Kmegtate@AOL.com

msmith

NURSING MADE INSANELY EASY!

3rd Edition

Sylvia Rayfield, MN, RN, CNS
Executive Officer, I CAN, Inc.

Loretta Manning, MSN, RN, GNP
Executive Officer, I CAN, Inc.

 ICAN, Inc. Publishing • Gulf Shores, AL

I CAN, Inc. Publishing, Gulf Shores, Alabama

P.O. Box 4409, Gulf Shores, Alabama 36547 • (800) 234-0575
www.icanpublishing.com

Editorial Assistant: Teresa R. Davidson
Cartoon Illustrations: Teresa R. Davidson, Greensboro, NC; Eileen
    Burke, Pass Christian, MS; Paulina Hanson, Words & Pictures;
    Jeanne Woods, Design Master, New Orleans, LA; Mitch Rubin,
    Rubin Art, Albuquerque, NM
Cover Design: Cheryl L. Quaid, Quaid Creative Projections, Gulf Shores, AL
Production: Linda Seaman, Patterson Printing Company, Benton Harbor, MI

Printed in the United States of America
ISBN 0-9643622-6-0
Library of Congress Catalog Card Number: 2001 135748

Nursing procedures and/or practice described in this book should be
applied by the nurse or healthcare practitioner under appropriate supervision
according to established professional standards of care. These standards
should be used with regard to the unique circumstances that apply in each
practice situation. Every effort has been taken to validate and confirm the
accuracy of information presented and to describe generally accepted
practices. However, the authors, editors, and publisher cannot accept any
responsibility for errors or omissions or for consequences from application of
the information in this book and make no warranty, express or implied, with
respect to the contents of this book. Every effort has been exerted by the
authors and publisher to ensure that drug selection and dosage set forth in
this text are in accord with current recommendations and practice at the time
of publication. However, in view of ongoing research, the constant flow on
information relating to governmental regulations, drug therapy, and drug
reactions, the reader is urged to check the manufactures information on the
package insert of each drug for any change in indications and dosage and for
added warnings and precautions. This is particularly important when the
recommended agent is a new or infrequently used drug. This book is written
to be used as a memory tool (A Visual Approach to Memory) for students,
graduates, and faculty. It is not intended for use as a primary resource for
procedures, treatments, medications, or to serve as a complete textbook for
nursing care. Copies of this book may be obtained directly from I CAN, Inc.
(see order form in the back of this book.)

ACKNOWLEDGMENTS

We wish to express our appreciation to both our families for their never ending support and love, while we developed this book.

- Randy Manning and Cheryl Quaid who have loved and supported us through our many books and all our other life endeavors.

- Our parents, Juanita Shera and Margaret Wright, who continue to believe we can do anything.

- The artists that take our words and ideas and interpret them into meaningful and sometimes hilarious images.

- Our contributors (students, teachers and friends) that see worth in our work and want to be a part of it.

- Our associates in Sylvia Rayfield and Associates, Inc., who make the words and images come to life when they present them in NCLEX reviews.

- Beverly Walker and Thom Maddox, and John and Clara Fults who jump through hoops with us to get our books to the nurses that need them.

Discovering new ways of thinking about nursing concepts and creative ways of helping learners to remember was the reason for writing this book. This is our 3rd edition of a book that has sold internationally and helped thousands of learners "get it". We are grateful to our contributors.

Julia Aucion, DNS, RN, BC
Associate Professor
Cookville, TN

Marie Bremner, DSN, RN, CS
Professor,
Marietta, GA

Jo Carol Claborn, MS, RN
Executive Director,
Nursing Education Consultants, Dallas, TX

Katherine Crawford, MSN, RN
Case Manager,
Shreveport, LA

Martha Eakes, MSN, RNC, CNA
Maternal-Newborn Coordinator,
Greensboro, NC

Shannon D. Foxworth, AD, RN
Florence, SC

Nancy K. Lovell, MSN, RN
Instructor,
Galesburg, IL

Alita R. Maddox, APRN, MSN, PNP-C
Educator,
Bossier City, LA

Karna C. McBrayer, BSN, RN
Educator,
Laredo, TX

Jackie McVey, PhD, RN
Tyler, TX

Vanice W. Roberts, DSN, RN
Assistant Dean,
Kennesaw, GA

Martha Sherman, MSN, MA, RN
Associate Professor (retired),
Asheville, NC

JoAnn Zerwekh, EdD, RN, CARN, CADAC, FNP
Nursing Education Consultants,
Dallas, TX

Dedicated with love
to nursing students
and nursing instructors.

PREFACE

A Message to Our Learners

This book was developed to make learning and life easier for student nurses and their teachers in registered and practical nurse programs, graduating nursing students preparing for exit exams, new graduate nurses preparing for NCLEX-RN® and NCLEX-PN® exams and other medical and allied health students that will find it useful.

Our experience with thousands of learners each year has helped us develop images and strategies that accelerate the learning process. The format is insanely easy! On the left page is the "bottom line stuff" about the concept. The image or memory tool is on the right page.

This 3rd edition has many additional tools to help you remember vital nursing concepts. We have added chapters on management, infection control and physical assessment at the request of our readers.

Many of the most important aspects of nursing are not easily illustrated in visuals. We think these unshown characteristics are a vital part of nursing: COMPASSION, CONSIDERATION, COLLABORATION, COMMITMENT, CALMNESS, CREATIVITY and COURAGE. We worked on this project with love and fun because we've been both student nurses and nursing teachers. We know the scope of your undertaking.

Sylvia Rayfield
Loretta Manning

I
CAN

Did is a word
 of achievement,
Won't is a word
 of retreat,
Might is a word
 of bereavement
Can't is a word
 of defeat,
Ought is a word
 of duty,
Try is a word
 each hour,
Will is a word
 of beauty,
Can is a word
 of power.

—Author Unknown

"THE IMPORTANT THING IN SCIENCE IS NOT SO MUCH TO OBTAIN NEW FACTS AS TO DISCOVER NEW WAYS OF THINKING ABOUT THEM."

Sir William Bragg

TABLE OF CONTENTS

*What we ARE communicates
far more eloquently than anything
we can say or do.*

PRIORITIZING

We want to introduce you to "MERRY MANAGER". She will be the nurse manager that will accompany you on your journey through out these first two chapters. As you can see by looking at her, she is positive both in her management style as well as in her thinking. She is outcome oriented and always attempts to understand the concerns of her nursing staff. "MERRY" is indeed one of those eagles that every nurse wants to emulate. Join us as we begin our journey through this "INSANELY EASY" and FUN book. Thank you for selecting this book for your journey! Let's get started with prioritizing nursing care.

Nurses must be able to make decisions regarding how to prioritize nursing care. Nurses are daily faced with the challenge regarding which client should be assessed (**FIRST**).

F   *FIND HYPOXIA*–When the nurse has several clients to provide care for, oxygenation is always an immediate concern. Hypoxia may be a result of cardiac or respiratory complications. Physiological changes such as vital signs, skin color, or capillary refill are a few of the assessments the nurse would anticipate. Another assessment the nurse may anticipate may be an increase in anxiety or confusion. When there was no alteration in sensorium prior to the current medical condition, this clinical change may strongly represent hypoxia!

I   *IMMUNOCOMPROMISED*–If there are 4 clients, none of which are hypoxic, but one client is receiving chemotherapy or is immunocompromised from another medication or medical condition, then this client should be evaluated first. The objective is to prevent infections from being transferred to the client.

R   *REAL BLEEDING*–A client that is hemorrhaging from a trauma, surgery, etc. is also a priority. This client will present with changes in the vital signs, skin color, temperature, urine output, etc. which will result in alteration in tissue and organ perfusion. BLEEDING is BAD for the client! Let's get on with the care!

S   *SAFETY*–Any client who is at risk for injury from increased intracranial pressure or confusion from delirium or dementia would be important to assess first. A toddler playing with a balloon would also be at risk for injury.

T   *TRY INFECTION*–If a client is septic with a high fever, and has an order for blood cultures and antibiotics, this client may be the priority to assess first. The priority for this client is to obtain blood cultures as ordered prior to starting the antibiotic therapy.

©2002 I CAN Publishing, Inc.

MERRY MANAGER is our STAR manager, because she has the qualities that we believe are so important in any manager.

S *STRENGTH* to grow, help and allow others to grow
T *THE "HAPPINESS FACTOR"* (comfortable in her own shoes, is not a victim and does not blame)
A *A VISIONARY* that can think "out of the box"
R *REACTIVE LAST*, proactive first

DELEGATION

The "DELEGATOR" delegates tasks but NOT responsibility. He tells his colleague how to be helpful to him. (*It is important to practice excellent communication skills or the colleague may become "stinky" like a skunk!*) Management issues are a part of the NCLEX® Test Plan. Delegating has always been a part of management, but the scope of practice laws vary from state to state regarding the meaning of delegation. These facts are a generalization and should generally keep the DELEGATOR out of trouble on the NCLEX®. Before we **TELL** someone to do something we know that we're usually legally responsible for the outcomes. These are the facts we need to know.

T *TAUGHT*–Has the individual been taught the skill, treatment or service?

E *EVALUATE*–Just because they have been taught how to do something doesn't mean they are competent to do it. Has their return demonstration been performed and documented?

L *LICENSE*–Does the individual have or need a license to do this task? Is it within their scope of practice?

L *LISTS*–What lists of standards of care (agency policies) are written regarding this task?

Remember–The DELEGATOR delegates the task NOT THE RESPONSIBILITY!

DELEGATOR

©1997 I CAN, Inc.

ANCILLARY PERSONNEL LIMITATIONS

LPNs and CNAs are key players in the current health care team. In order to delegate appropriately, the RN must be aware of their scope of practice. Since it will take more space than we have to review what both of these groups can do, let's review the **PART** of care the LPNs cannot do and the CNAs **CAN'T** do. This is based on our interpretations of the various Nurse Practice Acts as reflected across the United States of America.

LPN

P   *PLAN IN ISOLATION OF RN*–LPNs plan in collaboration with the RN. They will not do this in isolation of the RN.
PUSH IV MEDICATIONS–The current LPN standard is not to push IV medications.

A   *ASSESS INITIALLY*–LPNs will participate in ongoing assessments; however, the RN is responsible for the initial assessment.
ANALYZE–LPNs do not make nursing diagnosis or analyze the nursing care.

R   *REVIEW = EVALUATE IN ISOLATION OF RN*–The LPN is responsible for collaborating with the RN during the evaluation process.

T   *TEACH INITIALLY*–While LPNs may be involved in the teaching process, they are not responsible for initiating the teaching process. This is the responsibility of the RN. The LPN may reinforce teaching.

CNA

C   *CAN'T IRRIGATE A FOLEY*–The CNA should not conduct this intervention.
CAN'T MAKE CLINICAL DECISIONS–CNAs can make observations, but are not responsible for clinical decisions.

A   *ANTICIPATE CLINICAL CHANGES*–CNAs should never be accountable for anticipating client's clinical changes.

N   *NO INVASIVE PROCEDURES*–CNAs should not be accountable for any invasive procedures or specialized procedures.

T   *TEACH*–CNAs are not responsible for teaching.

ANCILLARY PERSONNEL LIMITATIONS

©2002 I CAN Publishing, Inc.

COST EFFECTIVENESS

"MERRY MANAGER" is responsible for managing both the quality of nursing care as well as the financial budget. It is imperative for her as well as all nurses to be cost effective. **SAVE** will assist you and "MERRY" in reviewing some strategies to achieve the outcome of cost effectiveness.

S   *STAFF*–When making assignments, the selection of the appropriate nursing personnel is a key component in being cost effective. If an LPN is able to provide the nursing care safely and efficiently, it is not financially wise to assign the RN to the same client.

A   *AVOID DUPLICATION*–This will also assist in providing cost effective care. For example, if a department has an unlicensed nursing personnel scheduled to run arterial blood gases to the lab, but the individual is only busy during the morning; it is wise to share this staff member with another unit and share in the cost.

V   *VIEW INFECTION*–"AN OUNCE OF PREVENTION IS WORTH A POUND OF CURE". Infections are expensive! Wash those hands and practice universal precautions.

E   *EDUCATE*–Discuss the budget with the nursing staff. (*An informed consumer is a smart shopper.*) AN INFORMED STAFF MEMBER CAN BE A SMART MANAGER!

COST EFFECTIVENESS

DISASTER PLAN

A disaster plan needs to be activated when there is a life threatening risk and a large number of clients must be evacuated from the hospital, assisted living units, etc. "MERRY" needs a way to remember which clients to remove first from the rooms. **ABC** will assist in organizing this information!

A *AMBULATORY*–The priority is to evacuate the largest volume of clients initially.

B *BED RIDDEN*–The bed ridden clients will be the next group to be evacuated from the rooms. Actually, the ambulatory group may be able to assist in getting this group evacuated more quickly.

C *CRITICAL CARE*–The last group of clients to be evacuated will be the critically ill.

The ultimate objective in a disaster plan is to evacuate volumes of clients. If the clients with numerous tubes and IVs are evacuated initially, this will slow the process down. Fewer clients will be safely rescued from the disaster.

DISASTER PLAN

LEGAL ASPECTS

DUE PROCESS–Hospitals, nursing homes, and other institutions where nurses practice have policies and procedures. For example, the little old lady climbs over her bedrail and falls on the floor. **Due process** is to pick her up, take her to x-ray, evaluate if anything is broken, complete and file an incident report, and notify her physician and family. If any of the steps identified as "**the due process**" are skipped, covered up, not charted or reported, there is a legal issue of negative proportions.

DECISION/ARBITRARY–The nurse's **decision** to refuse a family member visiting rights because she doesn't like their pierced nose and motorcycle jacket may be **arbitrary** and cause a legal issue.

DEPRIVATION OF PROPERTY–Nursing faculty that choose to give course outlines to all students during the first day of class, but refuse to share with the student who shows up the next day may be dealing with "**deprivation of property**".

DEPRIVATION OF CONFIDENTIALITY–The nurse that discusses one client with another may be dealing with a **deprivation of confidence**.

INTEGRITY TAKES US A LONG WAY IN KEEPING US OUT OF COURT!!!

LEGAL ASPECTS

UNIVERSAL PRECAUTIONS

Infection control is one very important nursing activity! A major problem in hospitals today is nosocomial infections. Something as simple as washing hands (**LATHERING UP**) can significantly decrease infections. Clients, family members, and health care providers must understand (**GIVE EXPLANATION**) the importance of infection control. Meticulous attention to aseptic technique when cleaning (**ORIFICES**) is effective in decreasing infections. **VERY SPECIAL HANDLING** of secretions, used equipment, needles, soiled linens, etc. is also important for decreasing infections. Nurses must remember when providing care that **EVERYONE MAY BE INFECTED**. The major concern for the nursing staff is the client who is infected and is unaware. When giving shots, starting IVs, or assisting with invasive procedures, meticulous attention must be paid to **SHARP** needles.

THE KEY TO PRACTICING UNIVERSAL PRECAUTIONS IS TO REMEMBER THE IMPORTANCE OF SAFELY HANDLING BLOOD AND BODY SECRETIONS!

In review, just remember **GLOVES** when practicing universal precautions.

G   *GLOVES*

L   *LATHER UP*

O   *ORIFICES*

V   *VERY SPECIAL HANDLING*

E   *EVERYONE MAY BE INFECTED*

S   *SHARPS*

GLOVES

G loves

L ather up

O rifices

G L O V E S

©2002 I CAN Publishing, Inc.

V ery special handling

E veryone may be infected

S harps

METHICILLIN-RESISTANT STAPHYLOCOCCUS AUREUS (MRSA)

Methicillin-resistant staphylococcus aureus (MRSA) is a common drug-resistant organism found in health care facilities. MRSA is difficult to control and treat. **Many cultures** must be done to identify the problem. Many different infections may be a result of this pathogen such as respiratory, skin, and urinary infections. As with other organisms, the nurse is not always able to tell that the client is infected. MRSA is spread primarily by direct and indirect contact. Occasionally it is transmitted through the respiratory and urinary tracts. Standard precautions will prevent the spread of MRSA, particularly in the skin and urine infections. If the MRSA is in the wound or urine, contact precautions are used. If the MRSA is in the respiratory tract then droplet precautions are used.

When incorporating Standard Precautions, **gown, gloves, and goggles** should be worn. Gloves must be worn when touching body substances, mucous membranes, nonintact skin, and items that are contaminated. They should be changed frequently after contact with infected items and material. If soiling is likely, then gowns should be worn. If body substances are going to be splashed, then a mask/face shield is indicated. Handwashing is always important to consider. Wash hands before and after care.

If MRSA is in the respiratory tract and droplet precautions are used, then a private room is necessary. There should be 3 feet of space between the client/resident and visitors. This can create a feeling of **social isolation** for the client. If it is necessary to transport the client in the hospital, then the client must wear a mask. The linen must be bagged to prevent contamination of self, environment, or outside of bag. Infectious trash must be discarded to prevent contamination of self, environment, or outside of bag. Masks/face shield for staff and visitors must be worn for individuals who are within 3 feet of the client. Noncritical care equipment should be limited to a single client. Hands must always be washed after completion of care and all of the gowns, gloves, etc. have been removed. Standard Precautions are always adapted in addition to the other specific types of isolation.

Since MRSA is such an **active infection**, it is imperative that meticulous attention is paid to isolation techniques. Remember, infection control is one of the top activities on the NCLEX-RN® test plan.

MRSA

M any cultures

MRSA

R equires gown, gloves, goggles

S ocial isolation

A ctive infection

FEVER

FEVER is the point where heat production exceeds heat loss. Our little digital thermometer is feeling badly. He has an ice pack on his head. His slippers indicate he is comtemplating a tepid bath.He is taking his acetaminophen or ibuprofen to prevent a rapid rise that may cause seizures. If none of these things work, the 101° Fahrehheit that can be tolerated can quickly rise to a dangerous level, especially at peak **FEVER** time late in the afternoon.

F *FAHRENHEIT* >100.4–100.8 (38° celsius)

E *ENDOGENOUS PYROGENS* reset the hypothalamic center

V *VOLUME NEEDS* increase secondary to heat loss (i.e., increased metabolism, shivering, sweating, evaporation, and vasodilation)

E *EVALUATE THE SOURCE VIA LABS*: CBC with differential, urinalysis, blood culture, and chest x-ray

R *RISK FACTORS*—viral or bacterial illness, environmental factors, tissue damage, biological agents, endocrine disorders

ALERT! GREATER THAN 107°F = DEATH OR IRREVERSIBLE BRAIN DAMAGE!

FEVER

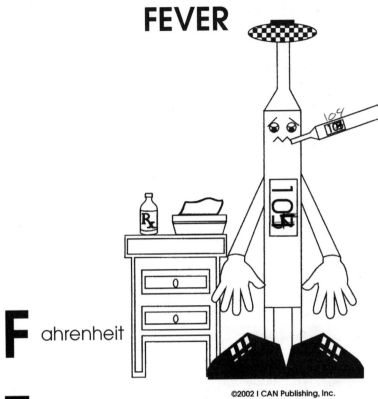

©2002 I CAN Publishing, Inc.

F ahrenheit

E ndogenous pyrogens

V olume needs

E valuate source via labs

R isk factors

BETA STREP

The 3 BEES help you to remember that with a **B STREP** infection it is wise to consider getting 3 cultures, administering 3 does of anti-infectives, and if momma BEE is pregnant she should be given her medication at the time of diagnosis as well as 2 more doses during delivery.

B *BETA-HEMOLYTIC STREPTOCOCCUS*– predominate causative agent in neonatal sepsis

S *SCREENING*– identify maternal carrier at 26–28 weeks gestation by vaginal swab

T *TREATMENT*–intrapartum with positive culture receives penicillin g chemoprophylaxis x 2 doses, neonates > 35 weeks gestation with effective treatment of mother are monitored for 48 hours, no early discharge, CBC with differential and blood cultures are drawn. If infant is symptomatic dual antibiotic coverage with ampicillin and gentamycin are recommended.

R *RISK FACTORS*– maternal GBS during pregnancy, < 37 weeks gestation, sibling with prior GBS infection, rupture of membranes > than 18 hours, intrapartum temp greater than 100.4° Fahrenheit or 38° celcius

E *EVALUATE INFANT* for s/s of sepsis usually appearing in first 48 hours–respiratory distress most common (apnea to mild tachypnea, labored breathing, increased oxygen requirements, mechanical ventilation), lethargy, poor feeding, hypoglycemia, temperature instability (hypothermia most common)

P *PROPHYLAXIS* should be given to mothers at time of diagnosis as well as 2 doses during delivery. If not accomplished due to precipitous delivery, treatment of the neonate should be considered.

B STREP

Beta-hemolytic streptococcus

Screening

Treatment ᵖⁿᶜ

Risk factors

Evaluate infant

Prophylaxis

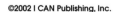

END OF LIFE

The end of life is a crucial time in our development that can be devastating or peaceful. Nursing can have a very positive effect on the client and the family during this time. While the nurse must always be cognizant of infection control, there is never a more important time than after death. Often unlicensed personnel prepare the body for the funeral home. Nursing responsibility includes teaching all persons safety in handling as the **BACTERIA DO NOT DIE WITH THE CLIENT.**

PAIN can usually be controlled. This is not the time to be worried that a client is going to get addicted to narcotics or sleep too much. If one pain medication does not work, it is the nurse's responsibility to evaluate this, bring it to the attention of the health provider in an assertive manner, and hopefully get an order for something that will work.

Many religions and cultures have very specific criteria about who can touch the body, rituals that must be performed and other **TREATMENT OF THE BODY AFTER DEATH**. The nurse's care and compassion will provide guidance towards honoring these traditions with respect. **ADVANCE DIRECTIVES** are very useful to family and clients. If clients have made their wishes known, there can often be more peace, less guilt and more guidelines for the Hospice nurse in assisting the client to die in dignity.

DEATH

D ying doesn't kill bacteria

E nd of life is often painful

A ggressive pain control

T he body treatment is vital

H ave advance directives

©2002 I CAN Publishing, Inc.

TOOLS OF
PHYSICAL ASSESSMENT

The tools of Physical Assessment are the most important in assessing, evaluating and monitoring the client's care. The appropriate tools include inspection, auscultation, percussion and palpation. Inspection is the use of the eyes to gather data. Careful observation can reveal clues about the client's respiratory system, musculoskeletal and neurological system, skin integrity, and the emotional and mental status.

Auscultation is the process of listening to sounds produced by the organs and tissues of the body. It is a clinical tool used most frequently to assess the heart, lungs, neck and abdomen. These sounds are characterized according to pitch, intensity, quality and duration.

Percussion is used for assessing the size, position and density of underlying structures. This technique consists of a sharp tapping that produces vibrations and subsequent sound waves. These sound waves are interpreted by the experienced percussor as air, fluid or solid material in an underlying structure.

Palpation is the use of hands and fingers to gather data through touch. The characteristics of body texture, temperature, size, shape and movement may be distinguished by different parts of the hands and fingers. The palm and ulnar surfaces are used to distinguish vibrations and the dorsal surface is best for estimating temperature. A bimanual technique uses both hands to entrap an organ or mass between the fingertips to better assess its size and shape.

Practice, practice and practice improve this skill.

TOOLS OF PHYSICAL ASSESSMENT

STETHOSCOPE

The stethoscope is indispensable for determining the sounds inside the body. The image on the next page will assist you in determining when to use the diaphragm or the bell of the stethoscope to hear the best sounds.

The diaphragm is used to hear high pitched heart sounds such as S_1 and S_2, murmurs of aortic and mitral valve regurgitation, pericardial, and abdominal friction rub sounds.

The bell is used to hear lower pitched heart sounds such as S_3, S_4 and a murmur of mitral stenosis.

THE STETHOSCOPE

DIAPHRAGM

H
I
G
H

Used to hear
HIGH-PITCHED
sounds
(lungs and heart)

S_1, S_2

BELL

O
W
E
R

Used to hear
LOWER-PITCHED
sounds
(heart)

S_3, S_4

VITAL SIGNS

Many learners indicate they have a hard time remembering the respiratory rate and the heart rate for the various stages of development. It in reality is quite simple! All you do is start with the neonate for your guidelines.

In order to determine the respiratory rate for the toddler, subtract 10 from the neonate, and the heart rate for the toddler can be determined by subtracting 20 from the neonate. Continue in this fashion for each of the stages. The next page outlines the averages to validate your figures.

Now, was that so hard?

VITAL SIGNS

Neonate

Respiratory 40

Heart Rate 140

Toddler (age 2–4)

Respiratory 30

Heart Rate 120

Child (6–10)

Respiratory 20

Heart Rate 100

Adult

Respiratory 12–18

Heart Rate 60–100

©1994 I CAN

CARDIAC SOUNDS

Cardiac sounds are one effective assessment for identifying alterations in the cardiaovascular system. S_1 is ordinarily auscultated over the tricuspid/mitral sites. It is heard in the beginning of the cardiac cycle (systole) and is described as the sound "Lubb".

S_2 is auscultated over the pulmonic/aortic site. It is heard at the end of the cardiac cycle (diastole). This sound is described as "Dubb".

S_3 is usually ascultated over the apex in the left side-lying position. It is heard in early diastole. The sound is described as "Ken-tuck-y". Hearing the S_3 may indicate heart failure, which also has 3 syllables (heart fail-ure).

S_4 can be auscultated over the apex in the left side-lying position. It is heard in late diastole and is described as "Tenn-e-see". Hearing the S_4 may indicate hypertension, which also has 4 syllables (hy-per-ten-sion). The PMI or Point of Maximal Intensity is usually ascultated midline at the 5th intercostal space.

CARDIAC SOUNDS

NORMAL

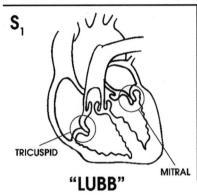

S$_1$

TRICUSPID

MITRAL

"LUBB"
Closure of
mitral and tricuspid valves

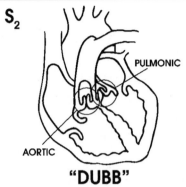

S$_2$

PULMONIC

AORTIC

"DUBB"
Closure of
aortic and pulmonic valves

ABNORMAL

S$_3$

Ken-tuck-y

**Heart Fail-ure
(3 syllables)**
Physiologic
(usually in children and young
adults)

S$_4$

Tenn-e-see

**Hy-per-ten-sion
(4 syllables)**

BREATH SOUNDS

Normal breath sounds have been organized into three categories based upon the intensity, pitch, and duration of the inspiratory and expiratory phases.

The bronchial sounds are heard over the manubrium (if heard at all). The expiration sounds are longer than inspiration sounds. They are louder and higher in pitch.
If these are auscultated anywhere other than the manubrium, they are considered to be abnormal and may indicate a complication with a lobar pneumonia.

The bronchovesicular sounds are heard often in the 1st and 2nd interspaces anteriorly and between the scapulae. The inspiratory and expiratory sounds are about equal in length. These sounds are intermediate. Differences in pitch and intensity are often more easily assessed during expiration. If bronchovesicular sounds are heard in other locations distant from what is listed above, then the air-filled lung may have been replaced by fluid or solid lung tissue.

The vesicular breath sounds may be auscultated over most of both lungs. Inspiratory sounds last longer than expiratory ones. Vesicular breath sounds are soft and low-pitched.

BREATH SOUNDS

TRANSMITTED VOICE SOUNDS

When the lung is normal and filled with air, spoken words are indistinct and muffled. The spoken "ee" is heard as "ee". Whispered words are faint and indistinct if heard at all. They are normally accompanied by vesicular breath sounds and normal tactile fremitus.

When these sounds go through an airless lung such as in lobar pneumonia or toward the top of a large pleural effusion, these spoken sounds (99, ee, 1,2,3) are louder and clearer (bronchophony). The spoken "ee" is heard as "ay" and whispered words are louder and clearer (whispered pectoriloquy). These transmitted voice sounds are usually accompanied by bronchial or bronchovesicular breath sounds and increased tactile fremitus.

Note: Remember to end in "phony" (phonics)-to understand clarity. Increase in clarity = consolidation!!

TRANSMITTED VOICE SOUNDS

©2002 I CAN Publishing, Inc.

Ego**phony** "ee"	=	"ay" sound
Broncho**phony** "99"	=	clarity of sounds
Whispered Pectoriloquy	=	clarity of sounds
"whisper 99 or 1,2,3"		

↓
Clarity of Sounds
↓
CONSOLIDATION

CRANIAL NERVES

This tool will help you to remember how some of the cranial nerves may be assessed.

3, 4, 6, makes my eyes do tricks!
Cranial nerves III, IV, and VI (oculomoter, trochlear, and abducens) assess extraocular movements.
Cranial nerve III is assessed by pupil constriction. Assess for pupils being equal and reactive to light.
Cranial nerve IV assesses eye movement.
Cranial nerve VI assesses lateral eye movement.

3, 4, 6, 8, how do we accommodate?
Cranial nerve VIII assesses hearing and balance. Check for hearing acuity.

3, 4, 6, 8

NEUROLOGICAL CHECKS

There has been a lot of mystery around "neuro checks." The bottom line here is that the client remains alert and oriented, the pupils are equal and reactive to light, and all extremities can move on command. Of course, you want to compare with the last time the neuro checks were done. Were the pupils equal and reactive to light? Were all extremities moving spontaneously and to command? PERL MAE is just lying there in her oyster with one side waving her arm and leg while the other side is limp. Observe that one of her pupils is larger than the other.

These assessments are crucial for any neurological client. Observe the subtle differences! For example, is the client more difficult to arouse than earlier? Your response to this change in assessments can mean the difference between a successful or an unsuccessful recovery!

PERL MAE

Pupils Equal Reactive to Light
Moving All Extremoties to command

©1994 I CAN

GROWTH AND DEVELOPMENT/HEALTH PROMOTION THROUGHOUT THE LIFE SPAN

From infancy to elderly there are major issues regarding health promotion that the nurse needs to review with the clients. The word SPINE will help you remember these issues.

S *STRESS MANAGEMENT* concerns clients throughout their lives. Children need to achieve various developmental milestones, which may be stressful during the growing process. As individuals age they must develop skill in adapting and coping to facilitate their stress management.

SAFETY is an important part of many clients' promotion of health. Safety includes anything from the toddler staying away from balloons to the elderly client watching for falls and drug/drug interactions.

P *PHYSICAL ACTIVITY* for the child to develop, activity to increase cardiovascular health and decrease osteoporosis are vitally important in health promotion.

I *INTERPERSONAL RELATIONSHIPS* are important to nuture. They prolong life and increase happiness. As the child grows into school age, their peers become increasingly more important in their life. During the working adult life, intimacy is an important developmental task.

N *NUTRITION* is of paramount importance throughout the lifespan to promote health and prevent disease. It is important that the adult takes in an average of 3 servings of milk, meat, vegetables, and fruits and 6 servings of bread or rice a day.

E *ENVIRONMENTAL SAFETY* is an important issue. We want to teach the importance of avoiding abuse, violence, poisoning, smoke inhalation, chemical spills and other noxious elements that put our life at risk.

GROWTH AND DEVELOPMENT/HEALTH PROMOTION THROUGHOUT THE LIFE SPAN

S tress
S afety

P hysical

I nterpersonal

N utrition

E nvironmental

©1997 I CAN, Inc.

INFANCY

Check out these kids and they will help you remember milestones for these ages. Developmental task is *TRUST* versus *MISTRUST* (Erikson).

0-3 months – Recliner is in the *RECLINING* position. His head lags. At two months lifts head and chest off bed. Totally dependent. Provide toys which are soft, cuddly and colorful.

3-6 months – *SITTER* – Starts rolling over. Six months of age can SIT for short periods of time leaning forward on hands. Birth weight may double at 6 months.

6-9 months – *BOUNCER OR CRAWLER* – Can pull self to a sitting position. They start bouncing so much that they bounce out and start crawling by 8–9 months. Everything goes in the mouth. Safety precautions!

9-12 months – *CRUISER OR WALKER* – Walks with help. This age loves to cruise around furniture. The birth weight may triple and length doubled (12 months). Shows stranger anxiety; clings to mother. Continues in solitary play and can entertain self for short periods of time.

INFANCY

First Three Months
Recliner (sleeps 20 hours a day)

3-6 Months
Sitter

6-9 Months
Bouncer or Crawler

9-12 Months
Crawler or
Cruiser

©1994 I CAN

TODDLER (1 to 3 years)

These children are "Into everything," have temper tantrums, and are called the "Terrible Two's". The typical words used with the toddler are "NO NO". Let's think of the opposite and consider PRAISING positive behavior. Refer to image for this explanation.

Notice in the image the child has a **PUSH-PULL** toy which is a favorite. Anything that will make them mobile so they can be **AUTONOMOUS**. These children like playing side by side (**PARALLEL PLAY**), but forget sharing!

The **R** is for the eyes because at bed time if certain **RITUALS AND ROUTINES** are not continued they will not close their eyes and go to sleep. Moral of that story is consistency! **REGRESSION** may occur during hospitalization. **PRAISE** appropriate behavior and ignore the rest. (*Easier said than done!*)

The **A** is for the body because toddlers are into **AUTONOMY**. They like to help dress and undress self. **ACCIDENTS** are a leading cause of death. They may have bruises on extremities from climbing and **EXPLORING** (**E** for feet). Keep poisons out of reach.

The **I** is for the arms, so they can be comforted by their parents. Allow parents to stay with child to decrease those **S**'s (tears) from **SEPARATION ANXIETY**.

ELIMINATION (toilet training) is one of the major milestones for the toddler.

PRAISE

P ush-pull toys
arallel play

R ituals & routines
egression

A utonomy versus shame & doubt
ccidents

I nvolve parents

S eparation anxiety

E limination
xplore

©1994 I CAN

POISON CONTROL

Tommy Toxin has crawled into trouble and ingested some substance that is toxic to his body. Mom should have **Syrup of Ipecac** around the house that will make Tommy throw up the material he has ingested. Once he has vomited, **Activated Charcoal** will act as an absorbent of the poison. If he has by chance swallowed any caustic or petroleum material (i.e., kerosene, gasoline), Ipecac will be contraindicated!

Calcium EDTA a chelating agent will probably be the most effective if Tommy ate paint or has lead poisoning. Our initial focus for Tommy would be ABC's (airway, breathing, and circulation). **"POISON"** will assist you with Tommy's plan of care.

P   *PREVENT* further absorption.   Decreasing absorption may be enhanced by syrup of IPECAC-in some facilities, gastric lavage has replaced Ipecac as the initial treatment. Activated charcoal may be given after gastric lavage or 30-60 minutes after induced emesis. Dialysis may be required if all else fails.

O   *OFF*–Shower or wash OFF substance if it is radioactive. If clothing is contaminated, take them OFF.
OUT–Take the toxic substance OUT of the body. If Tommy has pills in his mouth, take them OUT. Eye may need to be flushed OUT. Antidotes may be necessary for heroin or drug overdose. Ingested substances may be taken OUT of the body by emesis, lavage, absorbents, or cathartics.

I   *IDENTIFY* the toxic agent - Do an accurate history and identify any available poison.

S   *SUPPORT* the client both physically and psychologically. Parents may feel guilty in regards to their parenting role. SUPPORT is important!

O   *ONGOING* Safety education regarding poison control!

N   *NOTIFY* local poison control center, emergency facility, or physician for immediate care and advice regarding treatment.

Remember—The best solution to poisons is to keep them under lock and key.

TOMMY TOXIN

©1997 I CAN, Inc.

PRESCHOOL (3 to 6 years)

Preschoolers have imaginations that don't stop. The word that is characteristic of this stage is "Why?" They ask questions frequently. "Why is the sky blue?" "Why do dogs have tails?" Due to their active imagination, we have selected the word **MAGIC** to describe this stage of development.

M *MUTILATION*–They may fear mutilation. A typical statement is, "Cover my bo bo; don't let my blood run out!" Any invasive procedure is seen as mutilation (i.e., shot, I.V., enema, rectal temp., etc.).

A *ASSOCIATIVE PLAY*–They progress from parallel play to more cooperative play. An active imagination is great while pretending they are the nurse, doctor, teacher, etc. *ABANDONMENT*–Children are afraid of being left.

G *GUILT*–The feeling is that if I think something bad, the thought can cause a bad event to occur. This may cause guilt for the child.

I *INITIATIVE versus GUILT*–Child is very creative and may have an imaginary companion. Imaginative toys and devices are favorites.

C *CURIOUS*–Curious about factual information regarding the environment. They always ask, "Why?"

MAGIC

Mutilation

Associative play
bandoment

Guilt

Initiative
maginary playmate
magination

Curious

©1994 I CAN

SCHOOL AGE (6 to 12 years)

Can you see a big dimple in the chin of this child? When you look back over your school age photo albums, what do you often see in those pictures? Many of us see those crazy little **DIMPLES**!

This will help you to associate with this group.

D *DEATH*–The bogeyman will jump out from under the bed to get them. Be honest about funerals and burials. Encourage ventilation of thoughts and feelings.

I *INDUSTRY versus INFERIORITY*–"Chum" period. May enjoy collecting coins, cards, etc. May enjoy sports. IMMUNIZATIONS should be complete before entering school.

M *MODESTY*–More concerned with modesty and privacy. Pull those curtains and close those doors.

P *PEERS*–The younger children play mostly with their own sex. Older child is beginning to mix with opposite sex.

L *LOSS OF CONTROL*–Hospitalization is seen as a loss of control. Allow and encourage decision making.

E *EXPLAIN PROCEDURES*–Use terms they can understand.

DIMPLE

D eath

I ndustry versus Inferiority
mmunizations

M odesty

P eers

L oss of control

©1994 I CAN

E xplanation of procedures

ADOLESCENT (12 to 18 years)

Adolescents are usually seen in groups or at least in **PAIRS**. Let's think about **PAIRS** while we review some milestones for the adolescent.

P *PEER* group is very important. Select activities involving peers (i.e., games, table tennis, etc.). Remember, carefully assess the diagnosis. Individualize the plan if client is on bedrest or in isolation.

A *ALTERED IMAGE*–They don't want to be seen as being different. Peer pressure may create problems with pregnancy, sexually transmitted diseases (STD's), substance abuse, and motor vehicle accidents. Health Promotion programs should be developed to make adolescents aware of STD's, contraception, and the effect of drugs and alcohol on the body.

I *IDENTITY*–Adolescents may be struggling for a sense of identity. They are making important choices regarding college or career.

R *ROLE DIFFUSION*–Who are they and what are their goals? Educate families and schools regarding these struggles.

S *SEPARATION FROM PEERS*–Peer interaction may be encouraged during their hospitalization.

PAIRS

P eer group

A ltered body image

I dentity—Image

R ole diffusion

S eparation from peers

©1994 I CAN

IMMUNIZATIONS

Those immunizations! "Nurses think they are hot shots giving us babies those shots! Let me see if there is a way that I can delay getting these immunizations!"

I   **IMMUNIZATION STATUS** (what has been given before)

M   **MMR** made with eggs–do not give with allergy to eggs or neomycin

M   **MUST** be without fever

U   **UPDATE** with new vaccines available: Prevnar, a pneumoccal vaccine, in now on the market

N   **NEVER** give in gluteals (thighs and deltoids)

I   **IMMUNE SUPPRESSION** disqualifies

Z   **"ZEIZURE"** disorders must be controlled before administration

E   **EVALUATE** sites for local reaction

D   **DOCUMENT**– site, lot number, parental consent, and RN signature

If child is diagnosed with leukemia, HIV infection, or is receiving a high dose of steroids, wait 3 months after therapy has stopped. Measles vaccine is recommended for asymptomatic HIV-infected children.

IMMUNIZED

I mmunization status

M MR made from eggs

M ust be without fever

U pdate with new vaccines available

N ever give in gluteals

I mmune suppression disqualifies

Z eizure disorders must be contolled

E valuate sites

D ocument

©1994 I CAN

DIAGNOSTIC PROCEDURES

As you review diagnostic procedures in all areas of nursing, focus on some specific areas to maintain safety for your clients before, during and after any procedure. We want to **ACT NOW** to prevent any complications with these information-gathering procedures.

A   *ALLERGIES* are an issue because many diagnostic tests use dyes. Assess for allergies, especially with iodine and shellfish which have iodine in them, prior to any procedure that uses dye. After these procedures, fluids will be encouraged to flush the dye out of the body. Some examples of procedures requiring dyes include myelograms, cardiac catheterizations, computerized axial tomography (CAT Scans), IVP's etc. *Remember the geriatric client excretes dyes slowly. Use with caution.*

C   *CONSENT FORMS* must be signed. The client should be well informed of the risks and benefits of the procedures.

T   *TEACH* the client regarding his participation and the data that the test will provide.

N   *NPO* is required for many tests. Clients and ancillary staff must be aware of this.

P O   *SITION* is important during and after many procedures. This information should be part of the pretest education.

W   *WHAT ARE THE VITAL SIGNS?* –VS's are an excellent way to determine the client's reaction to a procedure, especially if dye has been used.

DIAGNOSTIC PROCEDURES

A llergies

C onsent

T each

N P O

p **O** sition

W hat are the vital signs?

DANGER SIGNS IN PREGNANCY

Visualize in your mind (or on the next page) a pregnant woman who is experiencing some complications in her pregnancy. Her car will not start, and she calls a cab to take her to the hospital. The word **CABS** will help you remember these complications.

C *CHILLS AND FEVER*–Indicative of an infection, and is never normal during pregnancy.
CEREBRAL DISTURBANCES–Headaches during pregnancy can indicate severe preeclampsia.

A *ABDOMINAL PAIN*–Abdominal pain (epigastric area) may be due to edema of the liver capsule and may indicate a convulsion is impending. A rigid, board-like abdomen during the last trimester usually indicates abruptio placenta.

B *BLURRED VISION*–Visual disturbances may indicate elevated *BLOOD PRESSURE* or a complication with severe preeclampsia.
BLEEDING–Early bleeding could indicate a miscarriage, abortion, ectopic pregnancy or hydatiform mole. Bleeding in the last trimester may be indicative of placenta previa or abruptio placenta.

S *SWELLING*–Edema especially in the periorbital and digital areas is indicative of mild preeclampsia. Watch for *SUDDEN ESCAPE OF FLUID* (rupture of membranes)!

CABS

C hills and fever
erebral disturbances

A bdominal pain

B lurred vision
lood pressure
leeding

S welling
udden escape of fluid

©1994 I CAN

PREGNANCY-INDUCED HYPERTENSION

This condition is specifically associated with pregnancy, preeclampsia and eclampsia. When you think about the priority nursing care with this disorder, think about **PEACE**. It is of paramount importance to provide a peaceful environment to prevent seizure activity.

P *PROMOTE BEDREST, QUIET ENVIRONMENT*–These are crucial. In severe preeclampsia, absolute bedrest and sedatives (Valium) are important.

E *ENSURE HIGH PROTEIN INTAKE*–Due to proteinuria, protein intake should be increased in the diet. Sodium intake should remain normal. Avoid diuretics.

A *ANTIHYPERTENSIVE DRUG*–Apresoline is a vasodilator that may be used to decrease the blood pressure. It's safe since it doesn't cross the placental membrane. Check maternal BP, pulse and FHR.

C *CONVULSION*–Prevent or control seizures. Administer IV Magnesium Sulfate. Have the antidote, calcium gluconate at the bedside for emergencies. Decrease the environmental stimuli.

E *EVALUATE PHYSICAL PARAMETER*–Evaluate for complications of magnesium sulfate toxicity.

PEACE

P romote bedrest, quiet environment

E nsure high protein intake (1g/kg/day)

A ntihpertensive drug: Hydralazine
   (Apresoline)

C onvulsions (Magnesium Sulfate)

E valuate physical parameters
   1. Blood pressure
   2. Urine output
   3. Respirations
   4. Patella reflex

©1994 I CAN

MAGNESIUM SULFATE TOXICITY

Magnesium Sulfate is the drug given to women to prevent seizures with the complication of pregnancy-induced hypertension (PIH). This medicine is a central nervous system depressant. The antidote is calcium gluconate. How can you remember the signs of too much of this medicine? Just remember that before a client has a seizure they may let out a loud **BURP**! (Do they do this in reality? Not usually; it is only a memory technique.)

Let me introduce you to Bonnie Burp. She has the following problems:

B *BLOOD PRESSURE DECREASED*

U *URINE OUTPUT DECREASED*

R *RESPIRATIONS DECREASED*

P *PATELLA REFLEX ABSENT*

Bonnie is predisposed to these side effects because magnesium sulfate is a central nervous system depressant. It acts by blocking the neuromuscular transmission.

MAGNESIUM SULFATE TOXICITY

B lood pressure decreased

U rine output decreased

R espirations < 12

P atella reflex absent

©1994 I CAN

NONSTRESS TEST–
OBSTETRICAL DIAGNOSTIC
TEST

The purpose of this test is to observe the *RESPONSE* of the fetal heart rate to the stress of activity.

Procedure requires approximately 30 minutes; mother is in semi-Fowler's position; external monitor is applied to document fetal activity; mother activates the "mark button" on the electronic fetal monitor when she feels fetal movement.

> *NONREACTIVE*
> *NONSTRESS*
> *NOT GOOD*
>
> *REACTIVE*
>   (Rate of heart is elevated in
>   response to stress of activity)
> *RESPONSE IS*
> *REAL GOOD* from nonstress test

NON-STRESS TEST

NONSTRESS
NONREACTIVE

©1992 Sylvia Rayfield & Associates

REACTIVE

RESPONSE IS
REAL GOOD

SIGNS AND SYMPTOMS OF LABOR AND DELIVERY

Would you agree with us if we say there is a fetus in the uterus wanting to be delivered into the **WORLD**? The fetus will go through the mechanisms of labor. There will be some signs that will indicate this process is imminent. The word "**WORLDS**" will help.

W *WEIGHT LOSS*–Nausea, vomiting, diarrhea and indigestion are responsible for this sign.

O *OBSERVE CHANGE IN SENSATIONS*–Since lightening, the mother may no longer have shortness of breath. Now she may experience some rectal pressure and an increase in the leg cramps.

R *RUPTURE OF THE MEMBRANES*–After membranes rupture, delivery should occur within 24 hours to minimize the risk of infection.

L *LIGHTENING*–This is when the fetus descends into the pelvis. Mothers will refer to this as their baby "dropping."

D *DILATION AND EFFACEMENT*–These are the most indicative signs that labor is pending. Dilation is when the cervix progresses from 0 to 10 cm. in diameter, and effacement is the thinning of the cervix.

S *SHOW BLOODY*–This is the expulsion of the mucous plug.

Show—
Bloody

Dilation and
effacement

Lightening

Rupture of the
membranes

Observe change
in sensation

Weight loss

©1994 I CAN

FETAL HEART DECELERATIONS

What is happening? As you can see on the next page, there is pressure on the head of the fetus. The difference in this *EARLY DECELERATION* in contrast to a *LATE DECELERATION* is that the onset, fall and recovery of the heart rate coincide with the onset, peak and end of the contraction. This does not indicate a problem and usually occurs during the active phase of labor.

LATE DECELERATIONS indicate a problem with utero-placental insufficiency. (Refer to **LATE DECELERATIONS**.)

VARIABLE DECELERATIONS are usually shaped like a V or a squared U. These may occur any time during the contraction cycle or may be nonrepetitive. The pathophysiology is cord compression. The nursing care is to change the position of the mother. If it lasts more than one minute, attempt upward displacement of presenting part. Mother may be placed in the knee-chest position or Trendelenburg position. This pattern may indicate a prolapsed cord. If this is the case, prepare for immediate delivery. To assist with fetal oxygenation, the nurse may give the mother oxygen.

DECELERATIONS

head compression

Early

normal

↓ start to end than ↑

Late

turn her

Cocaine
HTN, DM
abrupto

uteroplacental insufficiency

cord compression

Variable

looks like a U or V on a strip

LATE DECELERATIONS

The Fire Department has come to the rescue of **FETAL DISTRESS**, and is planning to put out the problem. First, however, they must **UNCOIL** the fire hose. What does a late deceleration look like and what does it mean? It is a uniform shaped dip. The onset coincides with the peak of the contraction with the recovery occurring at the end or after the end of the contraction. It indicates uteroplacental insufficiency. If the fire department does not do something soon, the fetus is going to get into severe distress.

C   *CHANGE POSITION*–Place mother in the left lateral position. For supine hypotension, change the maternal position.

O   *OXYGEN*–Administer oxygen to mother to correct the uteroplacental insufficiency. If **OXYTOCIN** is infusing, stop the infusion. This may be causing uterine hyperactivity resulting in uteroplacental insufficiency.

I   *IV FLUIDS*–Epidurals may cause dilation. Increasing hydration with IV fluids will increase the maternal blood pressure and the uteroplacental circulation.

L   *LOWER THE HEAD OF THE BED* and elevate the feet to increase perfusion to the uterus.

LATE DECELERATIONS

FETAL DISTRESS

FD

Reprinted with permission
©1994 Martha Eakes

Change position (<u>left side</u>)

Oxygen
Oxytocin—off

IV fluids

Lower head

ACTIVE PHASE OF LABOR

During the first phase of labor, the mother is extroverted, feels great, and is going natural childbirth all the way (until she gets to this second phase)! Now, life has changed, and she is down right **MAD**! During the active phase of labor, mother is 4-7 cm. dilated with contractions occurring every 3-5 minutes lasting for 30-60 seconds. This phase can last approximately 6 hours.

M *MEDICATION*–Have the meds ready! She may reconsider and have an epidural. Meds are not given in the first phase (Latent) because they may slow the progress of labor. They are not given during the third phase due to potential suppression of the neonatal respiratory status.

A *ASSESS*–Assessments include: vital signs, cervical dilation and effacement, fetal monitor, etc.
ANTICIPATE PHYSICAL NEEDS–Mothers will appreciate you sponging their face, keeping their LINENS clean and DRY. Assess bladder for fullness.

D *DRY LIPS*–Mouth gets dry and can crack. Provide oral care! Mom will love you for being so thoughtful. (It's the little things that really count!)

ACTIVE = 4-7 cm.

q 3-5 min. contractions
30-60 seconds duration

Medications

Assess
Anticipate physical needs

Dry lips—ointment
Dry linens

©1994 I CAN

PITOCIN

Pitty Pitocin, this pregnant woman, is slow to begin active labor, so the Doc decides to induce by using **PITOCIN**. Watch for those major side effects!

Visualize Pitty sitting in a row boat looking into a **PIT** watching the "TETANIC" sink into the "ocean" (**OCIN**). Complications of this drug are **TETANIC CONTRACTIONS**. Pitocin of course is a stimulant; so as Pitty watches the ship sink, her blood *PRESSURE* elevates! Just as a sinking ship takes in all that salty WATER, poor Pitty is left holding the excess fluid in her body (observe **INTAKE** and **OUTPUT**). She gets so nervous with all this happening that she goes into **CARDIAC ARRHYTHMIAS** causing Pitty's baby *OXYGEN* hunger and **FETAL HEART IRREGULARITIES**. This is so upsetting to Pitty that she gets *NAUSEATED* and *VOMITS* all over the row boat.

STOP THAT PITOCIN DRIP!!!!!!

SIDE EFFECTS OF PITOCIN

Pressure is elevated

Intake and output

Tetanic contractions *no longer than 90 sec.*

Oxygen decrease in fetus

Cardiac arrhythmia

Irregularity in fetal heart rate

Nausea and vomiting

©1994 I CAN

REGIONAL ANESTHESIA

Regional anesthesia is used to anesthetize one **REGION** of the body; the client may remain awake and alert throughout the procedure. The image used will assist in recalling nursing care for the different **REGIONS** of the body.

R *RESPIRATORY PARALYSIS* – Have ventilatory support equipment available. Avoid the extreme Trendelenburg position before level of anesthesia is set.

E *ELIMINATION* – Evaluate the bladder for distention. When the epidural is done on a pregnant woman, labor may be delayed due to bladder distention.

G *GASTROINTESTINAL* – Check when client last ate. Position to prevent aspiration. Antiemetics need to be available along with suction equipment.

I *INFORM OF PROCEDURE* – Does the client under-stand the procedure? Check for drug allergies, make sure legal permit is signed and have client empty bladder.

O *OBSERVE FOR HYPOTENSION* – Report B/P less than 100 systolic, or any significant decrease. Change client's position, administer oxygen and increase IV rate if client is not prone to CHF.

N *NO TRAUMA TO EXTREMITIES* – Support extremities during movement. Remove legs from stirrups together.

ANESTHESIA

Respiratory paralysis

Elimination

G I

Inform of procedure

Observe for hypotension

No trauma to the extremities

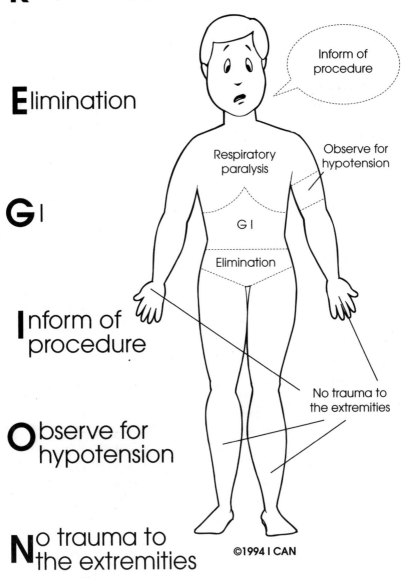

©1994 I CAN

TRANSITION PHASE

This is the last phase of the first stage of labor. Mother has gone from being MAD to being **TIRED**. She is now 8-10 cm. dilated and contractions are occurring every 2-3 minutes, lasting 45-90 seconds. This exhausting phase has duration of 1-2 hours. (MUCH TOO LONG; MOTHERS SAY!)

T *TIRES*–The mother continues to need a great deal of physical and emotional support.

I *INFORM OF PROGRESS*–Time drags on during this phase! The smallest progress is important.

R *RESTLESS*– "Please, can we get this show on the road?" (We were being polite; most mothers forget the word please at the peak of a contraction.) Support mothers with their breathing techniques. We don't want her pushing until she is totally dilated, so short panting breaths would be appropriate here.

E *ENCOURAGE AND PRAISE*–Go for it!

D *DISCOMFORT*–Mom is going to put all of her negotiating skills to work here in order to get the nurse to give her some pain medicine. No analgesics are given here because of the effect on the neonate's respiratory status.

TRANSITIONAL = 8-10 cm.

q 2-3 min. contractions
45-90 seconds duration

Tires

Inform of progress

Restless

Encourage and praise

Discomfort

©1994 I CAN

POSTPARTUM ASSESSMENT

If a parent's newborn is a son, they must "BUBBLE HE" during and after feedings. This will assist you with reviewing the postpartum assessment.

B *BREAST*–Assess for and prevent mastitis. Teach how to cleanse breasts and nipples. Support with breast feeding.

U *UTERUS*–Fundus should be firm and in the midline. Immediately after delivery, the top of the fundus is several finger breadths above the umbilicus. The fundus then descends into the pelvis approximately one finger breadth per day. Massage the fundus if it is boggy.

B *BLADDER*–Observe for bladder distention; it may displace the uterus. Diuresis occurs during the first two postpartal days. Evaluate for UTI.

B *BOWEL*–Stool softeners or laxatives may be necessary. By second or third day post delivery, normal bowel movements should occur.

L *LOCHIA* –Should not have foul odor. Rubra (dark red first 3 days), serosa (pinkish, sero-sanguinous 3 -10 days) and alba (creamy or yellowish after 10th day and may last a week or two).

E *EPISIOTOMY* –Observe for infection and healing.

H *HOMAN'S SIGN*– Observe for thrombophlebitis.

E *EMOTIONAL* –Support is a must!

POSTPARTUM ASSESSMENT

B reast *mastitis the mother needs to continue to breast feed.*

U terus *displaced to right or left means full bladder*

B ladder

B owel *stool softener Tucks*

L ochia

E pisiotomy

Reprinted with permission
©1994 Martha Eakes

H oman's sign *↑ for DVT*

E motional

postpartum blues should not last more than 2 wks

FOODS HIGH IN FOLIC ACID

Several conditions require a client to eat a diet high in folic acid. Some examples of these are: iron deficiency anemia, chronic alcoholism, pregnancy and malnutritional anemia. Here is a visual to help you remember those foods high in Folic Acid.

FOLIC ACID

Green Leafy Vegetables

SPINACH

Wheat Germ

FOLIC ACID

Liver

Legumes

FOODS HIGH IN IRON

What type of clients need to be on a diet high in iron? If you indicated any of the following, you are right. Clients with hemodilutional anemia who are pregnant, poor dietary intake of iron, surgery of gastrointestinal tract, problems with absorption and clients on IV therapy for 10 days or more need to be on a diet high in iron.

The foods which are high in iron are: organ meats (think about an organ that plays music), red meats, fish, green leafy vegetables, raisins (the California Raisin), sunflower seeds and legumes.

IRON

©1994 I CAN

FOODS HIGH IN PROTEIN

Foods high in protein can easily be remembered if you recall the jingle *Happy To Consume My Calories Sanely*. **H**amburger, **T**una, **C**hicken, **M**ilk, **C**ottage Cheese and **S**oy Beans are high in protein.

PROTEIN

©1994 I CAN

Happy	=	Hamburger
To	=	Tuna
Consume	=	Chicken
My	=	Milk
Calories	=	Cottage Cheese
Sanely	=	Soy Beans

FOODS HIGH IN POTASSIUM

An easy way to remember foods high in Potassium (K^+) is the **ABC Fruit** and **Veggie Plate**. Apples, Bananas, Cantaloupe (melons) and Citrus such as orange juice are high in K^+. Asparagus, Broccoli and Carrots are also high in potassium. Teach clients about the **ABC Fruit** and **Veggie Plate**, especially those clients who are taking diuretics.

Clients with severe burns, others who have hypersecretion of the adrenal cortex or on long term steroid therapy will benefit from these foods.

K FOODS = ABC FRUIT/ VEGGIE PLATE

©1994 I CAN

FRUITS	VEGGIES
Apples	**A**sparagus
Bananas	**B**roccoli
Cantaloupe	**C**arrots

FOODS HIGH IN SODIUM

The all-American **HOT DOG**–your way to remember foods that are high in salt (sodium). What is the first thing you must have for a hot dog? A wiener of course. Can't have a hot dog without a wiener and what is a wiener? It's processed meat in a tube that is high in salt.

Now, imagine walking through the delicatessen with us, looking up and seeing all of those tubes of meat hanging from the ceiling. Pressed ham, salami, bologna–all high in salt. Next we need a bun for the wiener. Of course, we put baking soda in our bread to make it rise (soda is salt). Next, comes ketchup which is processed tomatoes that are high in salt. Some folks will mess up a perfectly good hot dog with pickles! Did you ever make pickles? You throw cucumbers into brine (salt water). Those who have to have a chili dog, open a can of chili. Canned foods are usually high in salt. Then of course some of our German friends must have sauerkraut on their dogs which is also high in salt. So, to remember those foods high in sodium, all you have to know is **HOT DOG**!

FOODS HIGH IN SODIUM

©1994 I CAN

LOW RESIDUE DIET

Daddy had some sort of rectal surgery or diarrhea that makes it a necessity for him to sit on his pillow. Low residue diets are used to reduce fiber and slow bowel movements. Clients with Crohn's disease and colitis may benefit from this particular diet. Here's an easy way to remember the low residue diet.

L *LIMITED FAT AND FRIED FOODS*

O *ZERO MILK*

R *REAL FRESH FISH/ UNSEASONED GROUND MEAT*

E *EGGS BOILED*, not fried

S *STRAINED FOODS*

As you can see for yourself, this diet is NO FUN for Daddy!

LOW RESIDUE DIET

L imited fat

O zero milk

©1994 I CAN

R eal fresh fish/ground meat

E ggs boiled

S trained foods

THERAPEUTIC COMMUNICATION

Therapeutic interaction takes place when **TRUST** is established. Think of joining hands with someone special to you. The letters in **TRUST** help us remember the dynamics of therapeutic communication.

T   *TRY EXPRESSION* – Encourage the exploration of thoughts, perceptions, feelings, and actions. Use broad openings and ask open ended questions.

R   *REFLECTION OF WORDS* – Confirms to the person that you are actively listening. For example, "I am really mad at my mother for grounding me." "You sound angry because you were grounded."

U   *USE OF SILENCE* – Just sit and allow the person to make the next response.

S   *SETTING LIMITS* – What type of people may need to have limits set? People with personality and substance abuse disorders, affective disorders, children and spouses.

T   *TIME WITH CLIENT* – Taking time with the client allows them to know that you care even if they refuse to communicate.

TRUST

©1994 I CAN

Try expression

Reflection of words

Use of silence

Set limits

Time with client

EATING DISORDERS

Our friend, Hortense , has a major eating disorder. These disorders consist of anorexia nervosa, bulimia or pica. Hortense has bulimia, recurrent episodes of binge eating. Anorexia is an intense fear of becoming obese. Pica is persistent eating of substances without nutritional value such as clay for at least one month.

So what is the bottom line problem? It is a feeling of loss of control and low self-esteem. Let's look at **EATING** to help remember.

E *ENCOURAGE EXPRESSION OF FEELINGS* – Help identify angry and negative feelings and recognize her positive characteristics.

A *ALWAYS USE THE SAME SCALES* – Weigh daily immediately upon arising and following first voiding.

T *TO PROMOTE FEELINGS OF CONTROL*, encourage independent decision making.

I *INCLUDE DIETITIAN* and Hortense to determine calories required. Once the plan is developed do not discuss food or eating.

N *NO SIGNS OF MALNUTRITION* – Observe amount of food ingested. Offer support and positive reinforcement for improvements in eating behaviors.

G *GOAL* – To identify eating disorder and rule out physiological etiology. Assist Hortense to re-examine self and identify positive characteristics.

HAVE PATIENCE!

EATING DISORDERS

Encourage expression of feelings

Always use the same scales

To promote feelings of control

Include dietitian

No signs of malnutrition

Goal

©1994 I CAN

INTERVENTIONS FOR ANXIETY

ANXIETY! Welcome to nursing school! Would you agree? Perhaps we should say, "Welcome to life!" Before we can successfully help our clients deal with their anxiety, we need to remain **CALMER** ourselves.

C *CALM*–Create a comfortable, calm environment for relaxation. A quiet room with soft music may help enhance this feeling.

A *AWARENESS OF ANXIETY*– Identify and describe feelings. Modify stress producing situations.

L *LISTEN*–Listen to both client and to yourself. Implement "TRUST." Protect the defenses and coping mechanisms.

M *MEDICATIONS*–When all else fails, use those drugs. A memory tool for anti-anxiety medications is on the next page.

E *ENVIRONMENT*–Walking, crying, working and concrete tasks may help moderate anxiety. Safety is paramount if meds have to be used.

R *REASSURANCE*–Implement "TRUST."

INTERVENTIONS FOR ANXIETY

Calm

Anxiety-aware

Listen

Meds—Librium, Equanil, Atarax, Valium, and Serax

Environment

Reassurance

©1994 I CAN

ANTI-ANXIETY MEDICATIONS

Clients who are anxious may feel like they are going "**BATS**". These **BATS** will assist you in remembering these anti-anxiety medications.

B *BETA ADRENERGIC BLOCKERS* may be used for a rapid heart rate.
BENZODIAZEPINES such as alprayalam (Xanax), chlordiazepoxide (Librium), diazepam (Valium), lorazepam (Ativan) and others decrease anxiety by depressing the limbic and subcortical central nervous system.

A *ANTIHISTAMINES* such as hydroxyzine (Atarax) may decrease anxiety if the client is a potential abuser of benzodiazepines.

T *TRICYCLICS* and MAO inhibitors may be used for panic attacks.

S *SSRIs* (serotonin selective reuptake inhibitors) may be effective in managing anxiety.

ANTI-ANXIETY MEDICATIONS

B eta adrenergic Blockers
enzodiazepines

A ntihistamines—COPD or potential abuse of benzodiazepines

T ricyclics and MAO inhibitors for panic attacks

S SRIs

SYMPTOMS OF DEPRESSION

People that become depressed become very worried about themselves. They realize that they feel terrible and may feel trapped in these feelings. **IN SAD CAGES** will help you remember the symptoms and concerns of the depressed client.

I

N *INTEREST* is lacking in most everything. They may feel lethargic. Libido may be decreased and they are commonly apathetic. They may experience despair and become apathetic.

S *SLEEP* is hard to come by. They often have several hours of sleep and then awaken with the inability of going back to sleep. Real rest is often hopeless which may add to the depression. Some people may want to sleep all the time. They are so depressed they do not want to get out of bed.

A *APPETITE* is very often depressed. Food doesn't look good or taste good.

D *DEPRESSED* people can become very tearful. They no longer smile and have a "flat affect" or no expression on their face.

C *CONCENTRATION* is often lacking. They may not be able to do their jobs or maintain their relationships due to the depression.

A *ACTIVITY* is decreased. They may become "couch potatoes" and refuse to participate in routine activites. Exercise may be an activity that they can no longer perform.

G *GUILT* may bring a very negative view of self, world and future.

E *ENERGY* level is decreased. They may have a poverty of ideas and turn their aggressive feelings inward.

S *SUICIDE* precautions are mandatory. Maintaining a safe environment and negotiating a contract with them may be life saving.

SYMPTOMS OF DEPRESSION

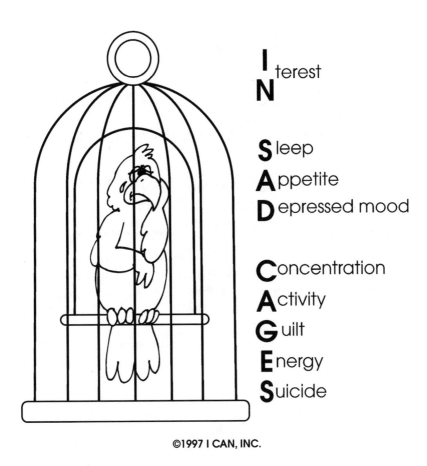

Interest

Sleep
Appetite
Depressed mood

Concentration
Activity
Guilt
Energy
Suicide

MANAGEMENT OF DEPRESSION

The depressed client is frequently seen alone and withdrawn from any meaningful social activities. The ultimate goal is to restore that socialization. Before that can be accomplished, trust with the nurse and eventually trust with a "**PEER**" must be established.

P *PREVENT SUICIDE*–The presence of a suicidal plan, including specifics relating to the method all indicate a potential risk. Remove harmful objects.

E *ENVIRONMENT*–A structured environment usually works best for the depressed client due to their impairment in decision-making. Encourage participation in activities and other simple tasks.

E *ESTEEM*–Encourage activities that promote a sense of accomplishment and enhance self-esteem. Encourage exercise and adequate rest.

R *RELATIONSHIP*–Encourage expression of feelings, thoughts or depressed feelings. Convey a kind, pleasant, concerned approach to promote a sense of dignity and self-worth in the client.

MANAGEMENT OF DEPRESSION

Prevent suicide

Environment

Esteem

Relationships

ANTIDEPRESSANT MEDICATIONS— TRICYCLIC ANTIDEPRESSANTS

Tina Tricycle is sitting on the curb because she is taking new antidepressants and should not drive heavy machinery. She may need to take her medication at night so she won't be too sleepy. Notice the number 3 on her tricycle. This will remind you that it takes approximately 3 weeks for the tricyclic antidepressants to achieve a therapeutic level. Her big **HAT** will help you remember some of the undesirable effects that she may experience while on this drug.

Tina must be taught that her compliance is vital to maintain a therapeutic level. She also must know that some herbs such as St. John's Wort may cause drug/drug interactions. Tina should not take MAO inhibitors while she is taking tricyclics.

Tina wants this medicine to improve her sad face and her interest in riding her tricycle.

TINA TRICYCLE

©2001 I CAN Publishing, Inc.

Hypotension
Anticholinergic
Tachycardia
Sedation

TINA

do not take MAO or st. John worts

T rimipramine

I mipramine

N ortriptyline

A mitriptyline

MONOAMINE OXIDASE INHIBITORS (MAO)

A few examples of these antidepressant medications are Marplan, Nardil and Parnate. They are given to inhibit the enzyme, monoamine oxidase, which breaks down norepinephrine and serotonin, increasing the concentration of these neurotransmitters. To assist you in reviewing the foods to stay away from while on these medicines, refer to the king on the next page or think of a tyrant (representing tyramine).

At 4:30 P.M. he goes into his study, and sits down to an ice cold mug of BEER, 2 glasses of WINE, and a platter of aged CHEESE. Later on in the evening, he goes into his dining room for a plate of LIVERS, home made steaming hot YEAST ROLLS, a bowl of FIGS, a glass of COLA, and a large piece of CHOCOLATE pie. In the middle of the table, there are 7 bottles of OVER-THE-COUNTER COLD MEDICINES. Tyramine is in most of these.

If the client takes tyramine (or any of these foods or meds), while on the MAO, it will cause a HYPERTENSIVE CRISIS. This will be characterized by increased temperature, tremors, tachycardia and a marked elevation in the blood pressure.

Watch for Strokes!

MONOAMINE OXIDASE (MAO) INHIBITORS

©1994 I CAN

BIPOLAR DISORDER

This psychiatric challenge is very well named. Our clown is interestingly dressed on one side and quite shabbily dressed on the other. Unless these folks are treated, their behavior is at opposite ends of the pole. Sometimes they will be so **UP** that they are manic, and other times they are so **DOWN** in the dumps that they're ready to kill themselves.

When they are **UP**, they may think they are Elvis or some other magnificent person. They may think this 24 hours a day. They don't have time to rest, eat or sleep. Try giving them finger foods and providing noncompetitive activities to decrease their hyperactivity. Setting limits, being firm and helping them stay on Lithium may be the best approach. Lithium works best when there is a sodium balance, so try to find them something to do besides play football which is sure to make them sweat. (Besides, this is competitive –Talk about hyper!)

When they are **DOWN**, it's hard to please them. Everything is negative, nothing is right. They still do not eat or sleep well because they are too depressed. Suicide is a common problem. Maintain Lithium at 0.5-1.5 meq/L. Report any assessment which will alter the sodium level.

GOOD LUCK!

BIPOLAR DISORDER

Mood elevated

A grandiose delusion

Need for sleep, eat ↓

Inappropriate

Clanging, loud, vulgar

Depressed

Out for suicide

Won't sleep, eat

Negative

Reprinted with permission
©1994 Nursing Education Consultants

Manic   Depressive

LITHIUM

Lithium is used for the **manic** episode in biplolar disorder. It acts to lower concentrations of norepinephrine and serotonin by inhibiting their release. Maintenance lithium serum levels should be between .5–1.5 mEq/Liter. Blood tests need to initially be done weekly. Maintenance blood **levels** should be done one time per month. Lithium should be taken the same time each day preferably with meals or milk. Do not crush, chew, or break the extended-release or film coated tablets.

Laboratory studies of the **thyroid** hormone and periodic palpation of the thyroid gland should be a part of preventive therapy. Report signs of hypothyroidism. Symptoms are reversible when lithium is discontinued and supplemental thyroid is provided.

Polyuria or **incontinence**, mild **thirst**, fine **hand tremors** or jaw tremors may occur in early treatment of mania or sometimes persist throughout therapy. Usually however, symptoms subside with temporary reduction of dose. A neuromuscular reaction is **unsteady** gait.

Encourage a diet containing normal amounts of **salt** and a **fluid** intake of 3 liters per day. Assess clients who are high risk to develop toxicity such as postoperative, dehydration, hyperthyroidism, renal disease, or those clients taking diuretics.

You will find LITHIUM on Monitoring Lab Values by the Magic 2s.

DRUG FOR MANIC CLIENT

Levels   .5 - 1.5   2 toxic

Incontinence

Thirst
Thyroid

Hand tremors

Increase fluids

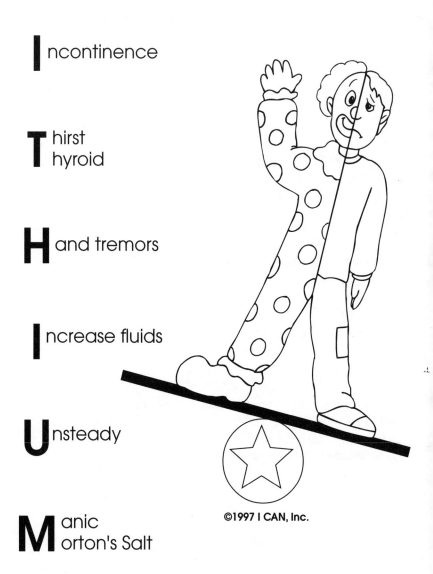

Unsteady

Manic
Morton's Salt

©1997 I CAN, Inc.

SCHIZOPHRENIA

The schizophrenic disorders are **HARD** to deal with. Their behavior is often maladaptive and involves alterations in thinking, moods, feelings, perceptions, communication patterns and interpersonal relationships.

The schizophrenic client has a **HARD** time with relationships and a **HARD** time with the establishment of trust. The word "**HARD**" may help you remember these concepts. It's **HARD** being schizophrenic and it's **HARD** (challenging) providing nursing care.

The nurse said to the person with schizophrenia, "It's time for lunch."

He said, "I'm DEAD, Dead folks don't eat."

She said, "It's time for meds."

He said, "Dead folks don't take meds."

She said, "Time for a bath."

You guessed it. "Dead folks don't bathe either."

How to prove to him that he was not dead? She had a great idea! She asked, "Do dead folks bleed?"

"Of course dead folks don't bleed," he answered.

She went after her needle and syringe and took some blood from his arm, held it up proudly and said, "SEE!"

He said, "I'll be damned, dead folks *do* bleed."

The moral to this story is that they cannot be reasoned with and the nursing care is **HARD**.

SCHIZOPHRENIA

©1994 I CAN

Hallucinations

Affect, ambivalence, autism, associative looseness

Relationship

Delusions

UNDESIRABLE EFFECTS OF ANTIPSYCHOTIC DRUGS

People that take antipsychotic drugs may have a different **STANCE**. They may shuffle their feet or have other unusual symptoms while taking these mood-altering drugs. **STANCE** will help you remember many of these undesirable effects.

S *SEDATION*, sleepiness and *SUNLIGHT SENSITIVITY* are common with these drugs. Often they are not able to drive.

T *TARDIVE DYSKINESIA* is an irreversible effect that changes the stance because it changes the head.

A *ANTICHOLINERGIC* effects can make the client's mouth dry and can cause constipation. *AGRANULO-CYTOSIS* is an undesirable effect. Report sore throats or signs of sepsis.

N *NEUROLEPTIC MALIGNANT SYNDROME* may occur.

C *CARDIAC EFFECTS* of orthostatic hypotension are common.

E *EXTRAPYRAMIDAL* effects such as pill rolling and akathesia may occur.

UNDESIRABLE EFFECTS OF ANTIPSYCHOTICS

S edation
unlight sensitivity

T ardive dyskinesia

A nticholinergic
granulocytosis

N euroleptic malignant syndrome
↓ LOC flex in BP

C ardiac arrhythmias (orthostatic hypotension)

E xtrapyramidal (akathesia)

©2001 I CAN Publishing, Inc.

ALCOHOLISM

One of the goals during the long-term rehabilitation is to assist client in identifying alternate coping mechanisms. "**COPES**" is the key in reviewing the priority nursing plans.

C   *COPING MECHANISMS* – Encourage client to develop alternative coping mechanisms other than alcohol to deal with stress. The client must be responsible for sobriety.

O   *ORIENT TO COMMUNITY RESOURCES* – Refer clients to available community resources such as Alcoholics Anonymous (AA), Alanon and Alateen. Abuse of spouses or children often occur while the client is drinking. Notify appropriate protection services for suspected spouse or child abuse.

P   *PLAN* may include antabuse. Antabuse is a drug used by a willing client as a deterrent that will make the client violently ill (flushing, hypotension and nausea and vomiting if he takes it and drinks alcohol). The nurse should always know when the client had the last drink before she administers this drug. Never administer any medications or substances with alcohol in them (i.e., cough syrup, mouth wash, shaving cream, etc.) while the client is taking antabuse.

E   *ENCOURAGE DIET* – Vitamin B complex is often used for the alcoholic client with delerium tremens and for the treatment of peripheral neuritis. Alcoholics often have avitaminosis because they drink instead of eat. Folic acid deficiency can lead to obstetrical complications.

S   *SEIZURES* – Delerium Tremens usually occur within 48 hours after cessation of drinking. Picking at the bed covers, tremors of hands, anxiety, nausea, hypertension and nightmares followed by seizures may cause an emergency.

ALCOHOLISM

©1994 I CAN

Coping mechanisms

Orient to community resources

Plan may include antabuse

Encourage vitamin B, folic acid

Seizures

DEMENTIA

"The Slow House of Alzheimer's" tells the story of "Poppa" who came to live with his son, but was so confused. The first night Son found Poppa a mile down the road in his pajama shirt and boxer shorts. He had fallen and his leg was bleeding. Poppa was "going to the house" (4 states away). To protect him, Son put a chair in front of his bedroom door, so that when he got up in the middle of the night he would be heard. Poppa would have gone nuts if he had been restrained. Barriers are much safer and more humane.

Son's wife could not wait to take Poppa to the cafeteria dining room so he could choose his own food, but Poppa stood there and stood there. Son's wife had to choose his food because decisions were impossible. The bathroom was a problem. Poppa had used the "out of doors" when he was a boy and his memory had regressed. It was easier to schedule his elimination than to embarrass the neighbors. Unfortunately the schedule was not always accurate and sometimes there were embarrassing wet clothes.

This story is a common one for people with dementia. **"The Slow House of Alzheimer's"** will help you remember the symptoms of **lost** and **wandering, confusion, decision difficulty, incontinence** and **confinement for safety**.

These changes are often progressive and irreversible. The cardinal rule for the geriatric population is do not push too fast (go slowly). It is important to reorient Poppa to the current **reality**. Objects such as clocks and calendars may help. Poppa's self-esteem may benefit through **reminiscing**. He may be able to recall events 10 years ago, but not 10 minutes ago. Poppa needs to be encouraged to remain **independent** as long as possible. Avoid dependency. Develop a plan for activities of daily living and remember **consistency** is important. As Poppa has illustrated, **safety** is very important. Due to sundowners and the increase risk of wandering and falling, **safety** precautions may become a high priority for these clients.

Remember–The difference between dementia (Alzheimer's) and delirium. Dementia is progressive and irreversible. Delirium or acute confusion state can result from sepsis, drug drug interactions, fluid and electrolyte imbalances, etc.

THE SLOW HOUSE OF ALZHEIMER'S

SAFETY CONFINEMENT

INCONTINENCE

CONFUSION AND DECISION DIFFICULTY

LOST AND WANDERING

©1997 I CAN, Inc.

LATER CHANGES IN DEMENTIA

Dementia is devastating to the client that knows something is "wrong" as well as heartbreaking to loved ones. The image on the next page will assist you in identifying some of the later changes in dementia. As you can see **APHASIA** is an issue with speech. They may not be able to talk or to understand. They may develop **APRAXIA** and lose their ability to perform purposeful activity. Sensory stimuli loss (**AGNOSIA**) may be common. The inability to remember certain items (**ANOMIA**) is frustrating and may make them angry. They may lose their memory (**AMNESIA**) and fail to recognize their spouse and children.

Dementia affects the client, the family and the caretakers. Remember, "caretakers die first". For this reason it is important that nurses help caretakers find support and relief from a demented loved one.

LATER CHANGES WITH DEMENTIA

APHASIA
SPEECH

ANOMIA
MEMORY OF ITEMS

APRAXIA
PURPOSEFUL ACTIVITY

AMNESIA
LOSS MEMORY

AGNOSIA
SENSORY STIMULI

COMBAT

Many people feel they put combat boots on the minute they get up in the morning, but we are referring to the client who is out of control. This may include folks that are real mad, manics, alcoholics, dementias and personality disorders just to name a few. It does not matter what the etiology is; the concept of "**COMBAT**" is still the same.

C   *CONTROL IMMEDIATE SITUATION*–Get their attention. Remove harmful objects. Maintain distance between self and client. Remain neutral.

O   *OUT OF SITUATION*–Remove client from the environment to de-escalate combative behavior.

M   *MAINTAIN CALM*–Do not hurry. Channel the agitated behavior.

B   *BE FIRM AND SET LIMITS*–Be consistent and prevent overt aggression.

A   *AVOID RESTRAINTS*–Use restraints as a last intervention.

T   *TRY CONSEQUENCES* –Positive consequences for positive behavior.

COMBAT

Control immediate

Out of situation

Maintain calm

Be firm/set limits

Avoid restraints

Try consequences

VISUAL CHANGES

The images on the next page will help you recall the major eye disorders. **GLAUCOMA** is described by clients as seeing halos around lights. Tunnel vision is another common complaint resulting from an increase in intraocular pressure. Loss of vision can occur. Glaucoma is chronic and a major cause of blindness.

CATARACT is a complete or partial opacity of the lens. This disorder is described as a decrease in visual acuity. Imagine you had on your sunglasses, and we took a paint brush and painted white paint on the outside of your glasses. Could you see out? Of course not. Is it painful? No. That is similar to cataracts.

RETINAL DETACHMENT is described as a sensation of having a veil or curtain over the eye. This disorder is sudden in onset. Some clients may experience an area of blank vision. Retinal detachment occurs from a separation of the two layers of the retina. When separation occurs, vitreous humor seeps between the layers and detachment of the retina from the choroid occurs.

MACULAR DEGENERATION is described as a blind spot in the center of the field of vision. Peripheral vision is retained but client is unable to read, drive, etc. There is no cure at this time.

VISUAL CHANGES

Glaucoma

Halo tunnel

Cataracts

Blurred

Retinal detachment

Curtain

Macular degeneration

BLACK SPOT

Black spot

SYMPTOMS OF
OPEN ANGLE GLAUCOMA

The image on the next page shows a big cup (optic) in a tunnel (tunnel vision). The client with open angle glaucoma may occasionally see halos around lights. They experience a loss of peripheral vision, which creates this tunnel vision. The good news is that this is a painless condition. The bad news is that glaucoma is one of the leading causes of blindness. Although this condition is not an emergency, we want to help the clients prolong the effects of vision loss with medication. See the next page.

OPEN-ANGLE GLAUCOMA

Occasionally see halos around light

Peripheral vision (gradually lose)
ainless
rogressive vision loss

Early stages asymptomatic
nlarged optic cup

Not an emergency

TUNNEL

©2002 I CAN Publishing, Inc.

MEDICATIONS FOR OPEN ANGLE GLAUCOMA

Clients with glaucoma will experience an increase in intraocular pressure. They may feel as if there is a **"BAHM"** (a bomb going off in their eyes). Our bomb on the next page is pointed down because this is the direction that we want the intraocular pressure to go while our client is using these medications.

MEDICATIONS FOR OPEN ANGLE GLAUCOMA

B eta blockers—reduces production of aqueous humor (Timolol Maleate)

A nhydrase inhibitor—reduces the rate of formation of fluid (Acetazolamide)

H yperosmotics—reduces the rate of formation of fluid (Mannitol)

M iotics—facilitates outflow

MIOTICS

Miotics are given to people who have an elevated pressure in the eye due to glaucoma. The word miotics has a **C** in it for *constrict*. As a result of the constriction from these drugs, there is an increased flow of the aqueous humor. Interestingly enough, many of the miotic eye drops contain the word **CAR**. **CARpine**, **CARbachol**, and **piloCARpine** are all miotics.

Notice the tag on our friend's car. He *"KANT C"* well due to his tunnel vision. Clients with primary open-angle glaucoma experience a gradual loss of peripheral vision which is described as "tunnel vision." *Isn't that EASY?*

CONSTRICT EYES: GLAUCOMA

MIOTICS

C
O
N
NO ATROPINE!!
S
T
R
I
C
T

©1994 I CAN

CARpine
CARbachol
pilo**CAR**

EAR DROPS

Aren't these guys great! They have been "mascots" on our marketing materials since 1991. They epitomize Accelerated Learning.

The ear canal changes as we grow. To be sure that ear drops can get down into the ear, we need to remember how to hold the ear when we're putting in those drops. Notice the word *adult* has a **U** in it for **UP**. Hold the adult ear **UP** and back. Notice that the word *child* ends in a **D**. Hold the child's ear **DOWN** and back.

WHEN INSTALLING EAR DROPS REMEMBER THAT THE EAR IS

ADULT
P

CHILD
O
W
N

SENSORY • 147

SIADH

Soggy Sid has SIADH (syndrome of inappropriate antidiuretic hormone), a condition that continually releases the
antidiuretic hormone (ADH). With increased ADH, the body
retains water and gets so Soggy that water intoxication may
occur.

Sid's cap is hiding his bandaged head from a head injury,
which is a major risk factor for SIADH. Due to his cerebral
edema, he is prone to seizures. Notice his limbs are small.
There is no obvious edema, yet he has gained weight in his
body. The intake and output record will document low urinary
output because he's keeping it all on board. The urine specific
gravity will be high. The serum sodium will be decreased
(dilutional). Limit Soggy Sid's fluid intake. He may be given
diuretics to assist with fluid excretion, especially if he has
respiratory or cardiac problems. Keep Soggy Sid's bed flat or
only slightly elevated. This position of his head will decrease
the secretion of ADH. Keep the neuro checks going. Soggy Sid
is in serious condition!

SOGGY SID

DIABETES INSIPIDUS

Due to a lack of pitressin excretion from the Pituitary gland, poor Fido is hunting every fire hydrant in town because he urinates a lot (polyuria). This loss of body fluids will cause him to be very dehydrated, have a low specific gravity in his urine and his coat to be very dry. To monitor Fido, the nurse will need to keep accurate daily weights and watch his vital signs.

Offer him plenty to drink and keep a watch on his specific gravity. This guy can get dehydrated in a hurry and must be watched closely.

DIABETES INSIPIDUS

PITUITARY

Dry

I + O, daily weight

©1994 Adapted from
Creative Educators

Low specific gravity

Urinates lots

Treat = pituitary hormone

r**E** hydrate

HYPERTHYROIDISM

GO GETTER GERTRUDE will help you remember the major symptoms of hyperthyroidism. Her last name, of course, is Graves. Graves' disease is the result of hyperthyroidism. One look at this visually stunning creature, and you can see how thin she is and how her eyes "bug out" (exophthalmus). Everything is running except her menstrual periods. Her HEART is running fast (increased pulse), her BLOOD PRESSURE is running UP, and her basal metabolic rate (BMR) is running, therefore the metabolism of drugs will be faster. She can eat a whole chocolate cake without ever gaining an ounce. She is running so much that she is cleaning out closets that don't need cleaning at 3:00 in the morning. Notice she is wearing short sleeves and pants because it takes a lot of energy to run, and she is hot all the time. While planning her nursing care, lower the room temperature and get rid of all those excess blankets. A quiet room will be great! Well-balanced meals (high in calories and vitamins) is a must. Due to the eye changes, protect cornea from drying. GO GETTER'S diagnostic tests would reveal an increase in the following reports: T3 and T4, protein bound iodine (PBI), BMR, and uptake of I 131. (Refer to **Hypothyroidism.**)

GO GETTER GERTRUDE

THYROIDECTOMY

The **BOW TIE** is around his neck because the hyperactive thyroid gland has been removed. Post-op can be a crucial period for these folks because they may *BLEED*. Often the blood collects behind the neck, being pulled by gravity if he is lying on his back. Place him in semi-Fowler's position to avoid tension on the suture line. Observe the *AIRWAY* due to potential swelling from being traumatized during surgery. Vocal chords may be swollen. Assess frequently for noisy breathing and increased restlessness. Evaluate *VOCAL* changes; increasing hoarseness may be indicative of laryngeal edema. If these people get into trouble they can lose their airway fast. It's advisable to have a *TRACHEOTOMY SET* available to open an emergency airway. The *INCISION* needs to be observed for swelling which can occlude the airway. Watch for normal wound healing. We don't want an infection. Evaluate calcium levels; parathyroids may have been damaged or accidentally removed. Since calcium potentiates the movement of electrolytes across the cell membrane and electrolyte balance is imperative for the heart cells to work, low levels could create an *EMERGENCY*. Have calcium gluconate available!

POST-OP THYROIDECTOMY

Bleeding

Open airway

Whisper

Trache set

Incision

Emergency

©1994 I CAN

HYPOTHYROIDISM

This vision of loveliness is **MORBID MATILDA**. Her last name, as you've probably guessed, is Myxedema (Hypothyroid). She has a slow deterioration of the thyroid function. It occurs mostly in older adults and five times more frequently in women than in men.

As you can see, Matilda has the family "bug-eyes" and she has no menstrual period like her sister Gertrude, but that's where the resemblance ends. (Refer to **Hyperthyroidism**.) Matilda is not thin. In fact, she can look at a piece of chocolate cake and gain weight. She had rather sleep at 3:00 in the morning than clean closets. She may also be sleeping at 3:00 in the afternoon because of her lack of energy. Her long pants and putting her hands in her pocket will keep her warm. Increasing the room temperature may be necessary.

Matilda will be placed on lifelong thyroid replacement, and will be on a low-calorie, low cholesterol diet to help with her weight loss. Morbid Matilda does not like these changes. She is definitely not a very happy camper!

MORBID MATILDA

DIABETES MELLITUS

FIDO, the diabetic dog, is exhibiting all of the signs and symptoms of hyperglycemia. Sugar is floating around in his blood stream because there is no insulin to take the sugar into the cells.

Since the cells are starving for lack of sugar, Fido is dreaming of food. He has a huge appetite. His food bowl in front of him remains empty because he keeps trying to feed those starving cells (POLYPHAGIA). The high sugar content in his blood is pulling fluid from the cells which makes him very thirsty (POLYDIPSIA). Since his kidneys are compensating by dumping extra fluid and sugar out onto the street (POLYURIA), he has totally wet down the fire hydrant. Look at Fido's pants! They don't fit any more. The sugar and the fluid that he has taken in have not gone into his cells, since there is no insulin to assist in crossing over into the cell. As a result, poor Fido has LOST WEIGHT. What medication would you plan to have available? Insulin of course. (Refer to **Hypoglycemia**.)

WHAT'S WRONG
WITH FIDO?

©1994 Adapted from Creative Educators

INSULIN

Do you have difficulty remembering the onset, peak, and duration of the various types of insulin? Let us help simplify this for you, so it will be easy!! In your mind it will be helpful to categorize the rapid, intermediate, and long acting insulin. The onset of the regular insulin is 30–60 minutes. The onset of humalog is < 15 minutes. If you can recall this time frame being real fast, then you will be able to remember the other insulins. For the intermediate insulin, multiply 60 x 2 and the onset is 60–120 minutes. For the long acting insulin, multiply 120 x 2 and the onset is 240 min.–320 min.

As you can see on caps on the next page, the peak has a general progression. Regular starts with a peak of 3 hours. Multiply 3 x 2 to get a peak of 6–12 hours for the intermediate insulin. As you can see the long acting insulin's peak is increased to 8–20 hrs. (remember 6 + 2 = 8). These will assist you in remembering the average peak action for your examination.

The duration of Humalog is 4 hrs. The remainder of the times are in increments of 6. The regular insulin's duration is 6 hrs. Multiply that by 3 and the intermediate insulin is 18–24 hrs. The long acting insulin has the longest duration of 36 hrs. See **HYPOGLYCEMIA** for insulin reaction.

Lantus is a long acting insulin. It has an onset of 1.1 hrs. There is no peak and it has a duration of 24 hrs.

Remember–Regular insulin is the only insulin which may be given IV.

PEAK TIMES FOR INSULIN

SHORT
Blue
ONSET 30–60 MINUTES
(HUMALOG: <15 MIN)

COMBINATION
yellow
ONSET 30–60 MINUTES
THEN 1–2 HOURS

INTERMEDIATE
Real
ONSET 60–120 MINUTES

LONG
green
ONSET 240–320 MINUTES

HUMALOG — PEAK 1 hr — DURATION 4

REGULAR — PEAK 3 hrs — DURATION 6–8

REGULAR/NPH — PEAK 2–4 hrs / PEAK 6–12 hrs — DURATION 6–8 / 18–24

NPH — PEAK 6–12 hrs — DURATION 18–24

LENTE — PEAK 6–12 hrs — DURATION 18–24   24 hours

P Z I — PEAK 8–20 hrs — DURATION 36

HYPOGLYCEMIA

People taking insulin may have hypoglycemic reactions. This is a fact. Some diabetics have them everyday; others rarely have this problem. Teach them the symptoms, so they recognize their situation. Some of the signs and symptoms to observe are they may get suddenly *TIRED* and run out of steam. *TACHYCARDIA* (rapid pulse) occurs as a warning. *TREMORS* or nervousness are other warning signs. They often become *IRRITABLE* and *RESTLESS*. They may mow anyone down in the coke line to get some food due to *EXCESSIVE HUNGER*. They know if they don't, they may be out! *DIA-PHORESIS* is common, and is an excellent guideline for determining if the client is asleep versus having a hypoglycemic reaction. If the client is unconscious, administer glucagon IV. Encourage them to eat carbohydrates or drink milk if they are awake.

*If ever in doubt of a diagnosis of hypoglycemia versus hyperglycemia, give carbohydrates–severe hypoglycemia can result in permanent brain damage.

Remember this jingle to help recall the differences:

*COLD AND CLAMMY MEANS YOU NEED SOME CANDY
HOT AND DRY MEANS YOUR SUGAR IS HIGH.*

Jingle reprinted with permission, NEC, Dallas, Texas

SYMPTOMS OF HYPOGLYCEMIA

Tremors
achycardia

Irritability

Restless

Excessive hunger

Diaphoresis
epression

© 1997 I CAN, Inc.

CUSHING'S SYNDROME

One look at **CUSHY CARL** and you see his problem. He has an overproduction of hormones from the adrenal cortex. As you see, he's holding a "twinkie." These people may have a HIGH BLOOD SUGAR. The bag of chips he is holding indicates his INCREASE in SODIUM resulting in fluid retention. Increase in volume naturally will ELEVATE the BLOOD PRESSURE. Watch that POTASSIUM level, it will have a tendency to DECREASE and we certainly do not want his heart doing any strange dances (arrhythmias). Cushy's fat face also let's us know he's holding fluids. His "buffalo hump" probably scares him enough that his blood pressure goes up even higher. The sore on his leg won't heal because of his high blood sugar. (Would we want to protect him from INFECTION? You bet!)

Put 2 and 2 together. Would we want to give a diabetic steroids? Not if we can help it. Sometimes there are no options, so if this is the case, monitor the blood sugar. Now we know that cortisone (steroids) will increase the blood sugar even higher, increase edema, and increase the risk for infection. With all of this going on, Cushy will indeed need some assistance with his emotional state.

We know we would! What about you?

CUSHY CARL

ADDISON'S DISEASE

ANEMIC ADAM, whose last name is Addison, is Cushy Carl's half brother.(Refer to **Cushing's Syndrome**.) The whole family thinks they have opposite characteristics. Adam has a disorder which is caused by a decrease in secretion of the adrenal cortex hormone.

Adam craves salt since he doesn't have enough. That is the reason he is out in the field at the salt lick. Hyponatremia has a tendency to cause low blood pressure. In addition, his potassium may be increased. He has hypoglycemia and complains of being tired and weak much of the time. This weakness is a cardinal complaint and usually is more severe in times of stress. Occasionally, Adam stays in bed. After his anorexia, nausea, vomiting and diarrhea, he is dehydrated and has a serious loss in weight. After all of this, who wouldn't be tired and weak? His skin has turned bronze, and it is not due to too much sun. This is caused by increased levels of melanocyte stimulating hormone (MSH). To prevent addisonian crisis, corticosteroids will have to be replaced.

ANEMIC ADAM

CYANOTIC HEART DEFECTS

Some folks have a hard time remembering which of those congenital heart defects are cyanotic versus which are acyanotic.

NO PROBLEM, just remember all congenital heart defects that begin with the letter "T" are cyanotic defects. Color the "T" on the next page blue to help you remember this easy concept.

FOUR T'S

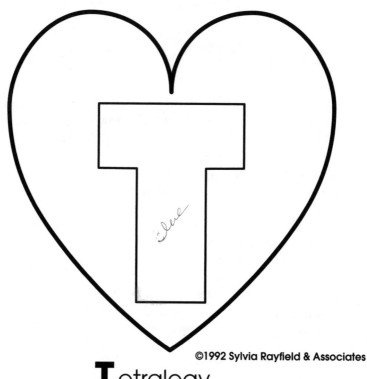

Tetralogy

Truncus

Transposition

Tricuspid

TETRALOGY OF FALLOT

Tetralogy of Fallot is often referred to as that complicated congenital heart defect that causes children to "squat" or "**DROP**" to the floor. When they get tired or out of breath, this position will decrease the amount of venous return to the heart. **DROP** will assist you in reviewing the four physiological defects with the heart in Tetralogy of Fallot.

D *DISPLACED AORTA* which allows unoxygenated blood into the oxygenated system causing cyanosis (overriding aorta).

R *RIGHT VENTRICLE HYPERTROPHIES* due to working so hard pumping against pressure. The more the heart muscle works the bigger it gets.

O *OPENING IN THE SEPTUM* is a "hole" that allows shunting of unoxygenated blood to mix with oxygenated blood (ventricular septal defect).

P *PULMONARY VALVE* partially closes making the right ventricle work, thus causing the right ventricle to hypertrophy.

These children are often small, tired, delicate and need surgery before leading a better quality of life. Teach parents to pace the child's activities, provide good nutrition to build strength and to renew themselves. Due to the challenges of these children, the parents need emotional support!

TETRALOGY OF FALLOT

©1994 I CAN

Displaced aorta

Right ventricle hypertrophy

Opening in septum

Pulmonary valve stenosis

HEARTS

This is to assist with remembering the nursing evaluation for an infant who has a serious defect requiring home care prior to corrective surgery. Think of a **HEART** since this is the location of surgery.

H *HEART MURMUR* – A murmur will be assessed especially with ventricular septal defects (VSD), atrial septal defects (ASD), and patent ductus arteriosus (PDA).

E *EVALUATE WEIGHT GAIN* – Due to their intolerance to suck well, they will have a slow weight gain. Some of these infants will be fed via a feeding tube because of their weakness.

A *ACTIVITY INTOLERANCE* – The infant fatigues easily. Conserve oxygen by anticipating their needs, so they won't cry.

R *RESPIRATORY INFECTIONS* – Due to pooling of blood in the pulmonary region, these infants have an increased frequency in respiratory infections.

T *TACHYCARDIA* – An elevation in the resting heart and respiratory rate are signs of hypoxia. Assess these changes carefully! They will give you a lot of information.

S *SUPPORT* – Allow family to grieve over loss of perfect infant. Foster early parent-infant attachment; encourage touching, holding and loving.

ASSESSMENTS FOR CONGENITAL HEART DISEASE

Heart murmur

Evaluate weight

©1994 I CAN

Activity intolerance

Respiratory infections

Tachycardia & Tachypnea

Support

HYPERTENSION

Catapres, a commonly used antihypertensive, is the name of our image to review RISK FACTORS. Just look at this gorgeous black woman. (Studies show that women of color have hypertension more often than other races.) See letters on the next page as you read below.

C People with hypertension may have small capillary hemorrhages in their eyes, blurred vision, and headaches.

A Nose bleeds could occur causing anxiety which leads to a further blood pressure increase.

T Carotid endarterectomies may be performed to prevent or relieve symptoms of a CVA caused from atherosclerosis of arteries in the throat.

A Her wide girth, obesity and hypertension go hand in hand.

P Pheochromocytoma and adrenal tumors can cause hypertension.

R Notice the feet; diabetics are known to have hypertension. Thickened toe nails and foot ulcers may result in gangrene.

E E stands for "Essential" hypertension (unknown cause). Early high blood pressure may have few symptoms.

S Sexual dysfunction may occur as a result from the medicines.

HEALTH PROMOTION IS A MUST!

CATAPRES

©1994 I CAN

REDUCE CARDIAC WORKLOAD

The car on the next page is carrying a **SPARE** "heart tire". The goal for nursing care is to decrease the stress and strain on the heart after a myocardial infarction. (*It is the same as our goal when we drive our automobile; we do not want our tire to be damaged. The spare tire never quite replaces the original.*) After a myocardial infarction, modification in diet and lifestyle are important nursing implications. Lifestyle and diet changes should include **restriction of sodium and saturated fat** and a reduction or avoidance of alcohol consumption. It is important to **provide a calm**, quiet environment and comfort measures to ensure effectiveness of pain medications. Immediately after a MI the nurse should allow the client time to rest between treatments, and limit visitors and extra activity. Cardiac **after load** can be decreased by medications such as vasodilators. These medications will relax the vascular smooth muscle, producing vasodilation of the arterioles which reduces the cardiac after load. Anxiety can increase the oxygen requirements significantly; therefore, it is important to **reduce anxiety** in the client's life and encourage **daily renewal and rest**. This is an important time in a client's life to learn new relaxation techniques. The ultimate goal is for the client to return to his/her activities of daily living and to live a happy, healthy, productive life!

REDUCE CARDIAC WORKLOAD

©1997 I CAN, INC.

S odium and saturated fat intake

P rovide a calm environment

A fter load reduced

R educe anxiety

E motional rest

ACE INHIBITORS

What is an ACE Inhibitor?

It lowers blood pressure by stopping the angiotensin converting enzyme (ACE) in the lung, which reduces the vasoconstrictor, angiotensin II. In other words, when you are playing cards, you may block the aces so your opponent will not win. This indeed will lower your blood pressure.

How do I remember all of these medications?

It's actually insanely easy!!! Remember they are pills and if you put an r after the p, you have a pril; these medications all end in **pril**.

Capto**pril**
Enala**pril**
Lisino**pril**
Fosino**pril**
Rami**pril**
Benzae**pril**

What do I need to evaluate?

1. Blood pressure - Since these medications reduce vasoconstriction, the pressure may go down too low. Observe for dizziness and/or tachycardia.

2. Some undesirable effects include an annoying dry cough, angioedema of the face, lips, tongue, and pharynx. Uncommon side effects include rash and taste disturbances.

3. Monitor for hyponatremia and hyperkalemia.

4. With Captopril, agranulocytosis or neutropenia may occur (ask about sore throats).

ACE INHIBITORS

 capto**pril**

 enala**pril**

 lisino**pril**

 fosino**pril**

 rami**pril**

 benaze**pril**

BETA BLOCKERS

Beta Blockers are a group of drugs that can be remembered using the acronym BETA. People taking these drugs may need TLC (tender loving care).

B *BROCHOSPASM* (so we don't want to give them to people with asthma or brochoconstrictive disease!)

E *ELICITS A DECREASE IN CARDIAC OUTPUT AND CONTRACTILITY.*

T *TREATS HYPERTENSION.*

A *AV CONDUCTION DECREASES* (short for treats arrhythmias, especially fast ones by decreasing the heart rate and cardiac output!)

REMEMBER–STOP BETA BLOCKERS
WITH BRONCHOCONSTRICTIVE DISEASE

T *TENORMIN* (atenolol) used for hypertension and angina (watch for renal impairment as this drug is renally excreted).

L *LOPRESSOR* (metoptolol) used for hypertension and angina (contraindicated in sinus bradycardia, 2nd or 3rd degree block, metabolized in liver and NOT renally excreted).

C *CORGARD* (nadolol) used for hypertension and angina (renally excreted, contraindicated in bronchial asthma, sinus bradycardia or 2nd or 3rd degree heart block).

NOTICE ALL THE GENERIC NAMES END IN "LOL"!

ROAD BLOCKS TO BETA BLOCKERS

©1997 I CAN, Inc.

CALCIUM CHANNEL BLOCKERS

This group of medications are often called "Don't Give a Flip Pills" by the clients who take them because that's exactly how they feel. Their blood pressure is lowered (calcium influx blocked), pulse is decreased, and if they move too quickly they get dizzy. They are much happier being a couch potato and taking life easy. A few examples of the calcium channel blockers include **Ca**rdizem, **Ca**rdene, Pro**ca**rdia, and **Ca**lan. Each of these common Calcium Channel Blockers have a **Ca** in them which makes it easy to remember! These medications should be administered with meals and milk. Some general undesirable effects of these medications include **constipation, bradycardia, peripheral edema, hypotension, dizziness, heart blocks, and worsening of CHF.**

Remember–Calcium Channel blockers should **not** *be given in clients who are in* **congestive heart failure** *or* **cardiogenic shock** *because they can decrease the heart rate too much.*

CALCIUM CHANNEL BLOCKERS

"DON'T GIVE A FLIP PILLS"

©1997 I CAN, Inc.

LOOP DIURETICS

Lou La Bell has been given a loop diuretic such as Lasix or Ethacrynate Sodium and is very **dizzy**. Her blood pressure has decreased too much after her excessive peeing. You would also feel as if you were spinning in a tube over the falls if you lost this much urine (volume). It may be very useful to teach her to get up slowly so she won't fall.

The life guard must blow his whistle in order to get her some assistance. She feels that the **ringing** in her ears just won't go away. **Dizziness** and **ringing** in the ears are major adverse reactions from loop diuretics.

A few other adverse reactions include: **hypokalemia, hypocalcemia (tetany), hyperglycemia, and hyperuricemia.** While **aplastic anemia and agranulocytosis** may occur, they are RARE!

Remember—Keep a close watch on blood pressure, potassium and calcium levels. Teach foods high in potassium and calcium. See ABC Fruit and Veggie Plate. Potassium supplements may be necessary.

LOU LA BELL

ATRIAL DYSRHYTHMIAS

If atrial fibrillation or atrial flutter occur greater than 48 hours in a client with normal cardiac function, diltiazem (Cardizem) is one agent that may be effective in controlling the **heart rate**. If the duration of the dysrhythmia is < 48 hours, consider the use of only one of the following agents for **converting the rhythm:** Amiodarone, Ibutilide, Flecainide, Propafenone, or Pocainamide. DC cardioversion. If the duration is > 48 hours or unknown, use antiarrhythmic agents with extreme caution. Avoid nonemergent cardioversion unless antiocoagulation or clot precautions are taken. For specific management refer to *2000 Handbook of Emergency Cardiovascular Care for Healthcare Providers*, p. 16, by American Heart Association. This management of delayed cardioversion and anticoagulation therapy are beyond the scope of this book.

In a client with an impaired heart (EF < 40% or CHF) and the AF > 48 hours duration, one of the following agents are recommended for controlling the **heart rate:** Digoxin, Diltiazem, Amiodarone. For this same client converting the AF in < 48 hours may be accomplished with Amiodarone. DC cardioversion. It the AF has persisted > 48 hours manage the anticoagulation and DC cardioversion. (*American Heart Association*)

Cardioversion may be indicated for heart rates >150 bpm with serious signs and symptoms related to tachycardia. Place the defibrillator/monitor in synchronized (sync) mode. The cardioversion may be painful due to the electric current going through the chest, therefore premedicate whenever possible.

Be prepared for the cardioversion to convert the rhythm to ventricular fibrillation. As our mothers always told us, too much of a good thing can be bad for us. Sometimes "stuff just happens"!

ATRIAL ACTIONS

Diltiazem (Cardizem)

C ✓ VS for bleeding
O
R do not in rayon.
A avoid ASA

I

G

©1994 I CAN

O

X

I

Now lie 'em down for cardioversion

Dig toxic Diggy
NV
Lalos

leggy Deggy

D. leve .5-2 toxic above 2

I. ↑ myocardio contractility

6. ↓ symptoms

HEART BLOCKS

A post graduate course in dysrhythmias will certainly provide more detailed information. The bottom line in heart blocks, whether it is 1st, 2nd, or 3rd degree, is when the **PACEMAKER** in the heart (SA node) is delayed or dysfunctional.

Drugs commonly used to treat this problem include **ATROPINE**, **EPINEPHRINE**, and **ISUPREL**. Atropine blocks the vagus nerve impulses on the SA node causing an increased heart rate. Epinephrine will increase bradycardia and increase myocardial contractility. Isuprel increases the ventricular rate and enhances cardiac conduction. This jingle will help in recalling **ISUPREL**:

ISUPREL IS A SOUTHERN BELLE.
SHE MAKES HEADS TURN AND HEART RATES GO UP!

According to the American Heart Association if the client is exhibiting serious signs and symptoms due to the bradycardia, then the intervention sequence would be as outlined below.

Atropine .5mg
Transcutaneous pacing if available
Dopamine
Epinephrine
Isoproterenol (Isuprel)

(For specific dosage, refer to *2000 Handbook of Emergency Cardiovascular Care for Healthcare Providers*, p. 14, by American Heart Association)

If the client begins experiencing a Type II second-degree AV block or Third-degree AV block, prepare for transvenous pacer. If the symptoms develop, use the transcutaneous pacemaker until the transvenous pacer is placed.

*If a pacemaker is inserted, teach client how to monitor their pulse which is an indicator of pacemaker function. Teach symptoms of pacemaker dysfunction and pertinent detail regarding "power" failure in permanent pacemakers. Provide a safe environment by eliminating all possible electrical hazards. Instruct these clients to wear medical identification.

HEART BLOCKS

©1994 I CAN

PACEMAKER

T   P
R   ISUPREL
O
P
I
N
E

VENTRICULAR FIBRILLATION

Adult Advanced Cardiac Life Support is not typically being taught by many nursing schools, as it is often considered post-graduate information. We have included parts of it, however, to give you 2 major ideas.

1. A general idea of what meds to expect to use during a cardiac arrest.
2. The material that often looks the most difficult can be reduced to INSANELY EASY!

Epinephrine or Vasopressin which would be a single dose (1 time only), Amiodarone, Lidocaine, Magnesium, Procainamide are several of the drugs used in ventricular fibrillation.

Defibrillate, Defibrillate, Defibrillate
Epinephrine, Defibrillate
Amiodarone, Defibrillate
Lidocaine Defibrillate,
Magnesium, Defibrillate,
Procainamide, Defibrillate

Refer to the next page for an easy way to remember these steps!

Defibrillate = Shock
Epinephrine = Everybody
Amiodarone = Amy
Lidocaine = Larry
Magnesium = Mama
Procainamide = Papa

Shock Shock Shock EVERYBODY SHOCK

Amy Shock—LARRY SHOCK
Mama Shock—Papa Shock

PULMONARY EDEMA

This condition is a result of too much fluid in the lung, both in the interstitial and in the alveolar spaces. Pulmonary edema results from severe impairment of the left heart function. MAD DOG COMES TO THE RESCUE!

M *MORPHINE* will decrease preload, allowing blood to pool in the extremities. As a result, the heart will not work as hard. A major problem is anxiety, due to feeling they are drowning in their secretions. Although morphine will decrease the anxiety, monitor for potential respiratory depression.

A *AMINOPHYLLINE* will decrease shortness of breath by expanding the bronchi. (Refer to Aminophylline Toxicity for more specific information.)

D *DIGOXIN* slows heart rate by increasing cardiac output. Hold med if apical heart rate below 60. Therapeutic level is 0.6–2.0 mg/ml; above 2.0 mg/ml is toxic. Signs of toxicity are anorexia, nausea, vomiting, headache, fatigue, bradycardia and photophobia.

D *DIURETICS*, especially Lasix dump the fluid overload through the kidneys. Monitor potassium level. Hypokalemia precipitates digitalis toxicity. (Therapeutic level of potassium is 3.5–5.0 mEq/L.) Daily weight will help evaluate the fluid loss along with an accurate intake and output record.

O *OXYGEN* is given to saturate red blood cells and provide more oxygen to the tissues. Oxygen is usually given via nasal cannula.

G *GASES* are evaluated to maintain pH, PO_2 and PCO_2 within appropriate limits. (Refer to **ACID-BASE**.)

PULMONARY EDEMA

Morphine

Aminophylline

Digoxin

Diuretics

Oxygen

Gases

©1993 Sylvia Rayfield & Associates

ACID-BASE

Draw a line down the middle of the right page. At the top of the left column put the numbers 7.35. At the top of the right column put 7.45. The normal blood pH should stay between these numbers. A pH below 7.35 indicates acidosis. A pH above 7.45 indicates alkalosis. Under 7.35 write CO_2 (body turns carbon dioxide to carbonic acid). Under 7.45 write HCO_3. Under HCO_3 write HCO_3 again and again. If we had enough paper we would write HCO_3 20 times because normal ratio of HCO_3 to pCO_2 is 20:1. The objective is to keep the pH between 7.35 and 7.45 which is done with buffer systems.

COLOR the van red. The red van represents the blood buffer system. Imagine the van driving through the arteries and veins of your body. When the pH gets below 7.35 (acidosis) the back van door opens, out jumps 20 little bicarbs, neutralizes the acid and gets back in the van to drive off! If the ph gets above 7.45 (alkalosis) the front van door opens, big powerful CO_2 jumps out, neutralizes and gets back in to drive off. This blood buffer is the first buffer system to respond to pH variations. The lungs follow by adjusting the respirations to regulate the CO_2. The third buffer system that helps maintain the pH are the kidneys.

7.35	7.45
CO_2	HCO_3
	HCO_3
	HCO_3
	HCO_3
	HCO_3

PO_2 90–100

PCO_2 45

HCO_2 22–26

©1994 I CAN

ACID-BASE STATUS

To determine acid-base status (respiratory or metabolic), picture yourself in Rome. You are on a playground with Phonetia (pH), Carbo (HCO_3), and Paco (pCO_2).

Phonetia and Paco hop on the see-saw and begin to play. Up and down, up and down. When the pH and pCO_2 are in opposite directions from "normal," the status is respiratory (respiratory = opposite).

Phonetia tires of playing with Paco and runs off to join Carbo who is on a swing. Both go up and both go down, always together. When pH and HCO_3 are either both up or both down, the status is metabolic (metabolic = equal).

pH > 7.45 = alkalosis
pH < 7.35 = acidosis

(Turn page for **COMPENSATORY MECHANISMS**).

Reprinted with permission from Creative Educators, Jefferson, LA

ACID-BASE

R espiratory

O pposite

M etabolic

E qual

Reprinted with permission
©1994 Creative Educators

COMPENSATORY MECHANISMS

(This will make more sense to you if you first refer to ACID-BASE STATUS.)

Compensation occurs in respiratory situations when Carbo gets mad at Phonetia for playing with Paco and hops on Paco's side of the see-saw! Imagine all three on the same see-saw. Compensation occurs in metabolic situations when Paco decides to crash the swinging twosome and hops on with Phonetia and Carbo. Now all go up or all go down.

Reprinted with permission from Creative Educators.

COMPENSATORY MECHANISMS

Respiratory

Metabolic

Reprinted with permission
©1994 Creative Educators

ACID-BASE

This referee is calling the shots in Acid-Base. He will help you remember if **ACID** or **BASE** is lost. Think, **A**bove the waist **A**cid is lost. **B**elow the waist **B**ase is lost. The stomach, above the waist, contains HCl (H^+ is an acid). HCl acid is lost during vomiting or when the client has a nasogastric tube. As a result, the client may develop a problem with alkalosis. When a client is hyperventilating, he increases the loss of carbon dioxide which also results in alkalosis.

The bowel below the waist contains alkaline substances which are lost during diarrhea. If alkali are lost, then the client may become acidotic.

There's a BIG exception here! Deep, prolonged vomiting will reach below the waist and lose alkaline intestinal juices resulting in a ketoacidotic state.

CALLING THE SHOTS IN ACID VS. BASE

ABOVE

A
C
I
D

BELOW

B
A
S
E

©1994 I CAN

SHOCK

When you think about the pathophysiology of shock, the classifications (except cardiogenic) have the common bond of decreased venous return (DVR).

HYPOVOLEMIC SHOCK (Hemorrhagic)—If an arm is cut off, that blood is certainly not returning to the heart. DVR! Another example of hypovolemic shock is the guy decides to roof his house on the 4th of July, and sweats out his volume, resulting in dehydration. Less blood to pump = DVR!

NEUROGENIC SHOCK— A severed spinal cord from a gunshot wound or fall allows blood to pool. Nerves have been cut; there is less venous constriction due to absent nerve stimulation. Spinal anesthesia and barbiturate overdose will cause the same response.

SEPTIC SHOCK (toxic)—An overwhelming infection; generally gram negative organisms will cause a dilation of the blood vessels resulting in a DVR.

VASOGENIC SHOCK (anaphylactic)—A DVR results from an antigen-antibody reaction with release of histamine. Blood that pools causes DVR! Less blood to pump = DVR!

(Refer to **Shock Interventions**.)

In contrast, CARDIOGENIC SHOCK is volume overload NOT volume deficit.

Shock
is
Decreased
Venous
Return

except Cardiogenic

HELP STAMP OUT SHOCK

S *SOLUTIONS* add volume and will increase venous return. Increase the rate. A combination of fluids, blood and plasma expanders (dextran, plasma and albumin) are commonly used. Watch for I.V.s with meds in them. We wouldn't want to turn up the I.V. rate of Pitocin!

H *HEMODYNAMICS* are a way to measure potential shock and evaluate interventions. CVP–(normal is a lucky 7) low CVP means DVR, (decreased venous return) or fluid deficit. Elevated CVP means fluid over-load as seen in cardiogenic shock. Low BP reading is one parameter that spells trouble.
Monitor it every few minutes. As meds are given to increase the BP, it will come up.

EARLY CHANGES	LATE CHANGES
Anxious	Coma
Heart rate elevated	Heart rate elevated and weak
Respirations elevated and deep	Respirations elevated and shallow
Skin cool, moist	Skin cold, clammy
Blood pressure no change	Blood pressure decreased
Normal skin color	Pale skin color

O *OXYGEN* will saturate those red blood cells and de-crease tissue starvation.

C *CHECK* the skin which is often cold and clammy.

K *KICK* up those feet and legs! There's a lot of blood volume in those legs. Elevate them and let gravity help increase venous return. Don't put the head down. Trendelenburg position may increase cranial pressure, ocular pressure and pressure on the diaphragm.

HELP STAMP OUT SHOCK

©1994 I CAN

Solutions

Hemodynamic changes

Oxygen

Checking

Kick 'em up

LUNG SOUNDS

Just breathing in and out makes a normal lung sound that can be heard with a stethoscope. Listen to both sides of the chest because the right side can have clear lung sounds while the left side can have "rales," "wheezes" or some adventitious breath sounds. Listen to the anterior (front) and posterior (back) sounds. How do we know if we hear rales? Rales, sounding like Rice Krispies doing "snap, crackle and pop," are most commonly heard around alveolar sacs more distal to the bronchial tubes. Rales have also been compared to the fizzling of a carbonated drink and are usually heard midway through the inspiratory phase. Wheezes are most often found over the midline or bronchi indicating constriction. Wheezes are continuous sounds, although they are heard more on expiration. Imagine hearing a whistle blow! This is similar to a wheeze.

The bottom line is that breath sounds should be clear and air should be heard moving on both inspiration and expiration. The key is to know what the normal is, so you can detect a difference.

ABNORMAL LUNG SOUNDS

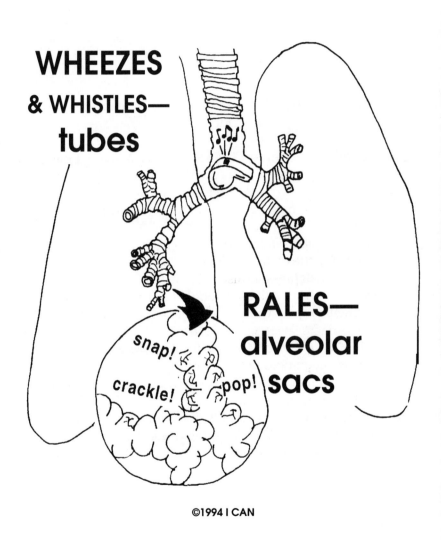

WHEEZES & WHISTLES— tubes

RALES— alveolar sacs

snap!

crackle!

pop!

©1994 I CAN

COPD

Chronic Obstructive Pulmonary Disease is referred to as emphysema. A major risk factor is cigarette smoking.

C   *COUGH* is chronic and nonproductive making it hard to breathe or rest well. A chest x-ray is often ordered to confirm the diagnosis and to look for pneumonia. Nope, one does not have to be NPO for a chest x-ray.

O   *OXYGEN* starvation demands oxygen. A good rule of thumb for the O_2 flow is 2-4 liters. High concentrations of oxygen depress the drive to breathe and cause respiratory distress. ABG's (arterial blood gases) are an excellent way to measure what's happening.

P   *PULMONARY FUNCTION TEST* shows a decrease in lung function possibly calling for postural drainage to reduce secretions and increase oxygen exchange.

D   *DON'T SMOKE* is probably excellent advice. Emotional support usually helps; nagging doesn't. Drugs and other stuff often given for **COPD** are included on the next page.

CHRONIC OBSTRUCTIVE PULMONARY DISEASE

©1994 I CAN

Cough

Oxygen and ABG's

Pulmonary function and postural drainage

Don't smoke

INTERVENTIONS FOR COPD (CHRONIC OBSTRUCTIVE PULMONARY DISEASE)

Since our primary objective for these clients is to enhance oxygen exchange, it makes sense to look at these medicines around the ABC's.

A   *AMINOPHYLLINE*–Relaxes the smooth muscle of the bronchial vessels. (Refer to Aminophylline Toxicity.)

B   *BRONCHODILATORS*–Epinephrine (adrenalin) is also used to relax smooth muscle of bronchials. Do not use if client has hypertension or cardiac arrhythmias.

C   *CHEST PHYSIOTHERAPY*–Help remove secretions from the lungs. (Refer to Postural Drainage.) *CORTICOSTEROIDS*–May be used to decrease inflammation.

D   *DELIVER OXYGEN AT 2 LITERS*–High concentrations of oxygen would eliminate the client's hypoxic drive and cause respiratory distress.

E   *EXPECTORANTS*–These will assist in decreasing the viscosity of the mucous.

F   *FORCE FLUIDS*–Fluids will facilitate the removal of secretions.

INTERVENTIONS FOR COPD
(A B C's)

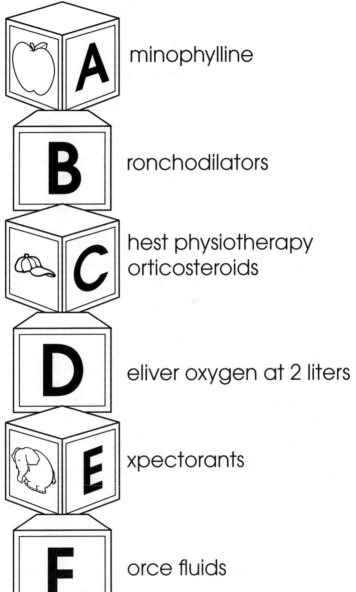

A — minophylline

B — ronchodilators

C — hest physiotherapy
orticosteroids

D — eliver oxygen at 2 liters

E — xpectorants

F — orce fluids

ASTHMA

***INFL* A** *MMATION*–Asthma is a chronic inflammatory process that produces mucosal edema, mucus secretion, and airway inflammation.

S *SYMPTOMS*–Wheezing, chest tightness, shortness of breath, cough. Use of accessory muscles in breathing. Symptoms of hypoxia and cyanosis occur late. Increased anxiety, restlessness, and exercise intolerance. Excessive sputum production.

T *TREATMENT* includes beta$_2$ adrenergic medications by nebulizer or metered dose inhalers. Epinephrine, antibiotics, (if an infection is present), broncho-dilators, expectorants. Inhalation of steroids to prevent edema. Supplemental oxygen for hypoxemia.

***IN* H** *ALERS* Inhalation of steroids to prevent edema. Beta$_2$-Adrenergic Agonists stimulate beta receptors in the lung, relaxes bronchial smooth muscle, in-creases vital capacity, and decreases airway resis-tance.

M *MECHANISMS*–Intermittent narrowing of the airway is caused by constriction of the smooth muscles of the bronchi and bronchioles. Excessive mucus production and mucosal edema of the respi-ratory tract are other mechanisms that contribute to asthma. Constriction of smooth muscle results in a significant increased airway resistance, resulting in trapped air in the lung. Emotional factors are also known to play an important role in precipitating an asthmatic attack for the child.

A *AVOID ALLERGENS*–Educate client regarding the importance of avoiding allergens that have been identified as precipitating factors resulting in an asthmatic attack.

ASTHMA

infl **A** mmation

S ymptoms

T reatment

in **H** alers

M echanisms

A voidance

AMINOPHYLLINE TOXICITY

Aminophylline (bronchodilator) is a wonderful and effective drug that relaxes and expands the bronchi reversing airway obstruction. This drug is commonly used in clients with problems such as: asthma, croup, chronic bronchitis and COPD.

Meet **AMILY TOXICITY** who received too much of this drug. We recommend that you stay out of her way! When she gets too much of this wonder drug, she **THROWS UP**! (Notice she has her hands covering her mouth.) Amily has an "A" on her shirt for "**hyperACTIVITY**". When the level gets high, Amily starts bouncing off the walls. The "**T**" on her shirt is for "**TACHYCARDIA**". Amily is so active that her heart rate must race (tachycardia) to keep up with her.

The therapeutic range for aminophylline levels is 10-20 mcg/ml.

*Keep your eyes open, and your assessments will tell you the story about the effectiveness of this drug. If signs of toxicity occur, report to the physician and check the TBL.

AMINOPHYLLINE TOXICITY

©1994 I CAN

Amily **T**oxicity

BETA$_2$-ADRENERGIC AGONISTS

MAX AIR, our friend on the next page, is holding several balloons to assist you in remembering some key points with these medications. Notice the balloons on the left are the clinical outcomes we expect from **MAX AIR**. Beta$_2$-Adrenergic Agonists stimulate the beta receptors in the lung, resulting in the relaxation of bronchial smooth muscles. This action results in an increased vital capacity which allows clients to breathe easier, resulting in the ability to blow up balloons.

Unfortunately, there are some undesirable effects that may occur while taking these medications. The balloons on the right will help you remember some key points. Tachycardia, irregular heart beat, hypertension, or cardiac dysrhythmias may occur. In addition to cardiac irregularities, other undesirable effects that may occur include nervousness, tremors, restlessness, insomnia, headache; nausea, or vomiting.

NOTE: For specific details about these drugs refer to *Pharmacology Made Insanely Easy* by Loretta Manning and Sylvia Rayfield. Specific details for ordering are in the back of this book.

BETA$_2$-ADRENERGIC AGONISTS

CYSTIC FIBROSIS

This little guy is a **"SICKER KID"**. His disease is inherited from an autosomal recessive trait. The exocrine glands that normally produce the enzymes lipase (digests fats), trypsin (digests protein) and amylase (digests starches) are not functioning normally. He's doing without a good part of his nutrition (about 40% of his food gets ingested). The other issue is that cystic fibrosis causes these enzymes to become so tenacious that they cause other problems. Organs affected by this disease include the lungs, pancreas, GI tract, and liver. **"Sicker Kid"** will assist you in remembering the major concepts in cystic fibrosis.

S *STEATORRHEA* (fat in stool) smelly stools with increased amount. *SWEAT TEST* indicating high salt content may be diagnostic. Adequate salt intake is important.

I *ILEUS-MECONIUM* may be present in newborns. The small intestine is blocked with thick mucous causing symptoms of intestinal obstruction.

C *CONSTANT HUNGER* because of poor food absorption.

K *VITAMINS K,A,D,E* (fat soluble) may be supplemented.

E *ENZYME* **(pancreatic)** *REPLACEMENT* is mandatory. Administer prior to meals and snacks.

R *REDUCE* dietary fat. Use **low fat** milk.

K *KEEP CALORIES UP.* Use **simple sugars** as a source of energy.

I *INFECTION* may be a way of life, especially respiratory infections due to pulmonary congestion. Administer oxygen and IV fluids to keep secretions thin.

D *DRINK PLENTY OF FLUIDS* to prevent dehydration and to keep mucous thin. DIET high in calorie, high protein, fats as tolerated or decreased, and increase salt intake.

CYSTIC FIBROSIS

S teatorrhea
  weat test

I leus-meconium

C onstant hunger

K vitamins

E nzyme replacement

R educe fat

K eep calories up

©1997 I CAN, Inc.

I nfection

D rink plenty of fluids

VENTILATOR CARE

This poor guy has found himself on a ventilator. To accurately evaluate the effectiveness of the vent, closely **VIEW** the client's **ARTERIAL BLOOD GASES**. Pressure should be maintained at the puncture site for a minimum of 5 minutes. After changing any ventilatory settings or suctioning the client, wait for 30 minutes to draw the ABG's. After procedures, carefully evaluate client's vital signs, pulse oximetry, color, etc., and check that **VENT** alarms are on. To determine the adequacy of air exchange, **EVALUATE** the **BREATH SOUNDS**. Look for equal chest movement, client's color and respirations. Calmly explain equipment and alarms to both the client and family. Ventilators are such a scary proposition that people become stressed. **NOTICE GI COMPLICATIONS** from potential **STRESS ULCERS**. The majority of clients will require a H_2 Histamine Antagonist.

The nurse must **TAKE NOTICE OF PRESSURE ALARMS** on the ventilator. An easy way to remember this information is that if the low alarm goes off, the priority of care is to check for a leak. To assist you in remembering this, _note there is a **l** in **low** and a **l** in **leak**_. If the high pressure alarm goes off, _remember **high** rhymes with **dry**_. The client may need suctioning or there may be water in the ventilator tubes. The tubes or client needs to dry out.

©1994 I CAN

View ABG's

Evaluate breath sounds

Notice G.I. complications (stress ulcer)

Take notice of pressure alarms

TUBERCULOSIS

INA has the typical signs and symptoms of tuberculosis including fatigue, weight loss, anorexia, chronic productive cough, night sweats, and hemoptysis (advanced stage). In order to help the *mycobacterium tuberculosis* **rise** out of her, there are several medications which may be prescribed. **"RISE"** will assist in remembering these medications.

R *RIFAMPIN*–This medication is most often prescribed with isoniazid (INH). The secretions (sweat, urine) may turn orange. Hepatitis may be a complication, especially in alcoholics. Rifampin should be administered once daily on an empty stomach.

I *ISONIAZID (INH)*–This is the primary medication used in prophylactic treatment of tuberculosis. Adverse reactions include hepatitis, and / or hepatotoxicity. Peripheral neuropathies can be prevented by pretreating with pyridoxine (vitamin B6). INH should be administered once daily on an empty stomach.

S *STREPTOMYCIN*–Two major adverse effects from this medication are ototoxicity and nephrotoxicity. Due to the susceptibility to cranial nerve VIII, this medication is generally avoided in the elderly. Use it with caution if clients have renal disease. Hearing must be evaluated frequently. Streptomycin may not be given po.

E *ETHAMBUTOL*–This medication is frequently administered with rifampin and INH. Assess vision prior to therapy to identify side effects of optic neuritis which may result in loss of central vision from this medication. Ethambutol should be administered once daily with food or meals to decrease gastric irritation.

INA TUBERCULOSIS

Drugs affect liver kidney
ring in ears
No contacts wear glasses
orange urine

antibodic
Monitor super infection
Evaluate liver & renal
Diarrhea — yogurt helps
Inform Dr of other meds

Cultures
Alcohol
Take full course of pill
Evaluate WBC, VS

©1997 I CAN, Inc.

FLUID VOLUME STATUS

The arrow indicates that fluid (plasma) volume decreases during dehydration. This will cause an increase in the sodium blood level above the normal range of 135-145 meq/L. The hematocrit will also rise (above 45%) due to the same principle.

The opposite occurs during pregnancy. Due to increased fluid (plasma) levels, the hematocrit and the serum sodium levels decrease. This dilution of the red blood cells is referred to as pseudoanemia. Evaluation of the serum sodium and hematocrit levels are excellent indicators of the fluid volume status. Several important nursing interventions for these clients include: daily weights, intake and output records, specific gravity evaluation of the urine, assessing the skin turgor, and lips and mucous membranes. An important assessment for infants regarding their fluid status is to observe if the fontanels are depressed or bulging.

This is an excellent tool to assist you in remembering the concept of the fluid volume status.

FLUID VOLUME STATUS

PLASMA
VOLUME

DEHYDRATION

Hct ↑

Na + ↑

FLUID SHIFTS

Fluid shifts are easier to figure out if you remember this nursery rhyme:

> "Mary had a little lamb and everywhere Mary went, the lamb was sure to go." Mary is salt (NaCl), and the lamb is water. Everywhere salt goes, water follows.

You may be asking yourself, how does this fit in with my nursing care? Frequently, we need to do health teaching for clients who are taking certain medications. The group that comes to our mind are the thiazides. Would we want these individuals eating a high sodium diet? Of course not! That would defeat the purpose for these diuretics.

Diuretics are given to remove fluid from the body. If we increase the sodium intake for these clients, they will continue to retain fluid. Everywhere salt (NaCl) goes, water follows.

FLUID SHIFTS

©1994 I CAN

"Mary had a little lamb and everywhere Mary went the lamb was sure to go."

RENAL PATHOLOGY

This system can be quite simple when you compare it to a water faucet and pitcher as we have on the image page. In the normal (healthy) faucet, the flow is great. There is no obstruction, and the filter is fine.

Notice in the **PRERENAL** diagram, there is decrease in the flow of water (urine). There is faucet (renal) ischemia–a decrease in the water pressure. Have you ever tried getting hot water out of the faucet while the dish washer is on? This can occur in the renal system from hemorrhage, shock, burns or decreased cardiac output.

In the **INTRARENAL** diagram, there is decreased output and some WBC's and protein which do not normally belong in the urine. This is due to kidney tissue pathology. In the faucet, it is as if someone came along and cut an opening in the filter on the spicket. This may be from glomerulonephritis, pyelonephritis, severe crushing injury, chemicals or medications.

In the **POSTRENAL** diagram, there is an obstruction in the water flow. This could be from the lime build up in the system which is causing a decrease in the free fluid. This is exactly what happens in the renal system. Some examples are: urinary calculi, benign prostatic hypertrophy (BPH) and cancer.

Remember to check renal function tests, BUN 10–20, creatinine .5–1.5. As the renal function decreases, these values will increase.

RENAL PATHOLOGY

Normal

50–60cc

Prerenal

<30cc

Intrarenal

Postrenal

BURNS

Berny has been in a fire, and as you can see, he is wrapped up like a mummy. Berny BURNS will help us learn burn care.

B *BREATHING*–Keep airway open. Facial burns, singed nasal hair, hoarseness, sooty sputum, bloody sputum, and labored respirations indicate TROUBLE!
   BODY IMAGE–Assist Berny in coping by encouraging expression of thoughts and feelings.

U *URINE OUTPUT*–In an adult, urine output should be 30 to 70 cc per hour, in the child 20 to 50 cc per hour, and in the infant 10 to 20 cc per hour. Watch the K^+ to keep it between 3.5–5.0 mEq/L. Keep the CVP around 12 cm water pressure.

R *RESUSCITATION OF FLUID*–Salt and electrolyte solutions are essential over the first 24 hours. Maintain BP at 90 to 100 systolic. One-half of the fluid for the first 24 hours should be administered over the first 8-hour period, then the remainder is administered over the next 16 hours. First 24-hour calculation starts at the time of injury.
   RULE OF NINE–Used for adults to determine burn surface area.

N *NUTRITION*–Protein and calories are components of the diet. Supplemental gastric tube feedings or hyperalimentation may be used in clients with large burned areas. Daily weights will assist in evaluating the nutritional needs.

S *SHOCK*–Watch the BP, CVP and renal function.
   SILVADENE–For infection.

REMEMBER THESE PEOPLE ARE AFRAID AND NEED SUPPORT!

BURNS

Breathing
Body image

Urine output

Rule of nine
Resuscitation of fluid

Nutrition

Shock
Silvadene

©1994 I CAN

CARE OF CLIENT AFTER MASTECTOMY

Have you ever had a chicken without a breast? Well, this may be a first for you. Meet "Ester the breastless chicken." Ester had a mastectomy due to cancer. She has a family history with both her mother and sister having breast cancer. She refused to have the recommended mammogram every 1 to 2 years after she turned 40.

After her mastectomy, no **BLOOD PRESSURES** or lab sticks were done on the affected side. She maintained the affected side in an **ELEVATED** position. Each joint was to be elevated and positioned higher than the more proximal joint to promote drainage. Ester met some wonderful women from **REACH FOR RECOVERY** who provided her with support. She was given pamphlets to read and phone numbers of some contact people who also had a mastectomy. After they left, she started her **EXTENSION** and **FLEXION** exercises. Squeezing a ball is a great exercise. **ABDUCTION** and **EXTERNAL** rotation should not be the initial exercises. Ester was taught how to do a SBE (self breast examination) once a month. The nurse recommended that she do it while she was taking her shower. The staff encouraged Ester to discuss her fears, concerns and anxieties in order **TO PROMOTE A POSITIVE SELF IMAGE.**

CARE OF CLIENT AFTER MASTECTOMY

BP—not on affected side

Reach for Recovery

Elevate affected side
xtension and flexion
    exercises—initially
    (squeeze a ball)

Abduction and external
    rotation should not
    be initial exercise

SB E—once a month—
    about one week after
    period

To promote a positive self image

©1994 I CAN

MENOPAUSE

MINNIE wakes up nights, throwing off those covers and finding herself wet with sweat from a hot flash. She reaches for her estrogen (premarin) with one hand since it will help control these night sweats and her heart shaped fan with the other. Her fan will cool her down, and it is heart shaped because during this time in her life she may wear her heart on her sleeve. She can be very sensitive and moody during menopause and small comments hurt her feelings. The estrogen will also improve Minnie's lipid profile and will decrease risks to her heart. (Refer to Josephine Bone-A-Part for more detail regarding estrogen.)

Vaginal BLEEDING seems to increase at menstrual period times and MINNIE must always be prepared with "supplies" because she can never tell when that period will show up. Excessive bleeding leads to ANEMIA and now she's got to take iron along with her other drugs, herbs and teas that reduce these "NO FUN symptoms".

Remember—This "PAUSE" is not a brief time in one's life and cannot be fixed quickly. Often symptoms persist for 3+ years!

MINNIE PAUSE

BENIGN PROSTATE HYPERTROPHY

The poor guy who has his "tubes" squeezed tightly due to an enlarged prostate gland will likely find himself going to surgery for a transurethral resection of the prostate (TURP). Prostatic tissue is removed through a resectoscope, so the urethra can once again pass urine easily.

When the guy comes back from surgery, he will likely have a triple lumen tube in his bladder to maintain continuous bladder irrigation (CBI) or Murphy drip. The *TUBE* will provide for *URINARY OUTPUT,* but it will contain bright *RED DRAINAGE*. If you see pieces of clots in the tube, it's time to increase the CBI to wash out the clots. Retained blood *CLOTS* may cause hemorrhage and we do not want that to happen! Unfortunately CLOTS may also cause bladder *SPASMS* that hurt. Belladonna and opium suppositories (B&O) are often ordered to help relieve the spasms. If the client complains of pain, evaluate the urinary drainage and make sure the catheter is patent.

Obstructions most commonly occur in the initial 24 hours due to clots in the bladder. Overdistention of the bladder can precipitate hemorrhage as well as bladder spasms.

TURPS

Tubes

Urinary output

Red drainage

Pieces of clots

Spasms

©1994 I CAN

SAFETY WITH RADIUM IMPLANTS

"How do you feel today" is adopted from Sue Crow's book *Asepsis, The Right Touch,* an excellent down to earth book on infection control. Let's assume that the character in the bed has a radium implant.

We want to plan our nursing care from afar! When you are in very close proximity to the client who has a radium implant, you get almost as much radiation as they do. Talk to them from as much DISTANCE as you can manage. Except when giving direct care, attempt to maintain distance of six feet from the source of radiation. Plan your care, so that you are in close proximity for the shortest period of TIME.

Some institutions provide lead SHIELDING; generally not necessary if time and distance principles are observed. Remember, these clients will get lonely because they are on bedrest and can't leave their room. *Be sure they can reach the telephone and the call light!*

EXTERNAL RADIATION

Sammy Shade is receiving external radiation for cancer. This source of radiation is directed toward the area of the tumor and draining lymphatics. He is likely to experience *SEVERE NAUSEA AND VOMITING, HEMATURIA and DIARRHEA.* Meticulous oral hygiene is important to decrease complications associated with vomiting. Antidiarrheal medications, low residue, high protein and a bland diet will decrease complications of diarrhea. Notice, Sammy has no hair on his head, very little on his face and probably none in his pubic area. Sammy will need help to cope with changes in his body image due to *ALOPECIA.* He may decide to wear a wig or turban. Sammy needs to pat, not rub, hair dry after shampooing to avoid excessive handling of brittle hair. Ice packs to the scalp may reduce hair loss. *ANEMIA* is a common side effect of therapy. Maintain adequate rest in between scheduled activities. Evaluate Sammy for signs of hypoxia. Encourage a diet high in protein, vitamins and iron. Assess for signs of infection and bleeding. External radiation is prone to *DRY THE SKIN* particularly *EVALUATE* the site of radiation. This site may remain photophobic, so let's advise Sammy to remain in the *SHADE.*

EXTERNAL RADIATION

S evere N & V

H ematuria

A lopecia
A nemia

D iarrhea

©1994 I CAN

E valuate skin for redness/dryness

TREATMENT OF ULCERATIVE COLITIS AND CROHN'S

Cathy Crampy has inflammatory bowel disease. She is bent over with the *CRAMPS* due to the inflammation. This is treated with steroids and a low fat and low fiber diet. Poor Cathy has her legs together to hold in that *DIARRHEA*. She is taking some antidiarrheal medications to decrease this problem.

Her *PAIN* is being relieved through her diet, *ANTICHOLIN-ERGICS* and corticosteroids. Cathy may be NPO to decrease bowel activity; FLUIDS are introduced gradually. She will receive IV fluids and may even require hyperalimentation to restore the deficiencies.

Sulfasalazine (*AZULFIDINE*) is one of the *ANTIMICROBIALS* used to prevent exacerbations.

Her MEALS are modified to correct the deficiencies. She is on a high protein, high caloric and high vitamin diet. Cathy may live a very stressful life. She is always a day behind her deadlines.

COUNSELING will help her to identify how this life style can contribute to this condition. Emotional *SUPPORT* will assist Cathy Crampy in decreasing the stress in her life and help her to learn "To slow down and stop and smell the flowers in life."

CRAMPS

Control diarrhea *high fiber diet*
Control inflammation

Relieve pain
Restore fluid

Anticholinergics → *I can't see*
Antimicrobials *pee, spit, shit*

Meals—correct *TPN*
   nutritional deficiencies

Psychological counseling

Support emotionally/coping

©1994 I CAN

COLOSTOMY

Clients with ulcerative colitis, Crohn's disease or other disease process in the lower gastrointestinal tract may require surgery that brings fecal elimination to an opening on the outside of the abdominal wall.

Connie Colostomy says that her colostomy is just like her **ANUS**.

A   *ABLE* to regulate her stool through regular irrigations; therefore a colostomy bag is not required. Irrigations should be the same time frame daily.

N   *NOT* watery. The stools are formed and do not leak on her clothes.

U   *U* can do all you can do without the colostomy. Some foods will liquefy stools or cause noisy problems.

S   *SWIMMING* is OK! Showers and tub baths are also acceptable.

This is probably NOT the case for Connie's friend ILLE who has an ileostomy.

Ille's stool is liquid. Bags are attached to the skin and skin breaks down easily. She must be taught about cleaning, removing the adhesive that holds the bag in place and cleanliness of the bag. She is usually not able to regulate the ileostomy because it is watery. She may lose fluids and electrolytes and need replacement. Some foods may also cause noisy (flatus) and "smelly" problems for Ille, which is embarrassing and hard to control.

Remember–Both Connie and Ille will have to live with these ostomys. The nurse's best approach is psychological support and education. They will need support through excellent therapeutic communication. The more they know about caring for themselves, the more "normal" they can be.

CONNIE COLOSTOMY

CONNIE COLOSTOMY

ILLE OSTOMY

©1997 I CAN, Inc.

PEPTIC ULCER DISEASE

Old **PUD** is a fine specimen of a man. He's standing there tapping his foot waiting impatiently on that bus, smoking his cigarette with a vengeance and checking to see if it's time for another NSAID (Nonsteroidal Anti-inflammatory drugs may cause GI bleeding). Just the kind of behavior that might precipitate peptic ulcer disease. When you think ulcers (except stress ulcers), think pain. Imagine a drop of hydrochloric acid on your open hand! First, the hand will hurt or burn, and once the acid has eaten the skin away, the hand will bleed. If the hand could be protected by a glove (food or drugs) the HCL might not eat through enough to bleed.

Drug timing is important in preventing this pain and bleeding. Generally, use anticholinergics before meals. (Refer to **Anticholinergics**.) Tagamet and zantac may be given with or after meals. Consider coating the stomach lining with the "white chalky stuff" such as maalox, titrilac, gelusil, or amphojel 1 hour after meals. Avoid giving within 1 to 2 hours of other medicines. Remind clients on sodium restriction to check the labels for sodium content. Amphojel, titralac, and digel have high sodium content. These clients will also need assistance in dietary modifications.

The Heliocobactor Pylori (Helicopter) organism may be responsible for PUD.

ULCERS

Pain

Ulcers bleed

Drug timing

Reprinted with permission
©1994 Nursing Education Consultants

GASTRIC REFLUX

As you can see, *GERD* is holding his stomach due to his problem with gastroesophageal reflux disease (GERD). He is also covering his mouth due to his discomfort with regurgitation of fluid and food particles. *GERD* is experiencing **REFLUX** of the stomach and duodenal contents into the esophagus leading to a spectrum of clinical manifestations predominated by inflammation of the esophagus.

REFLUX is most often related to inadequate relaxation of the lower esophageal sphincter (LES) that allows reflux of gastric acid and pepsin into the distal esophagus. Agents such as alcohol, benzodiazepines, calcium channel blockers, chocolate, peppermint, and narcotics cause LES relaxation.

REGURGITATION can be decreased by weight reduction if client is obese. The head of the bed may also be elevated. Alterations in the amount of **FOOD** eaten at one serving can also be effective in decreasing reflux. *GERD* should avoid large meals and sit upright 30 - 60 minutes after eating. *GERD* should **X** out carbonated beverages particularly 3 hours prior to going to bed. **ESOPHAGEAL SPASMS** may be relieved by avoiding agents that cause LES relaxation as indicated in the previous paragraph. As you can see, *GERD's* **LIFESTYLE** must be modified.

Remember *GERD* must manage this reflux, so he doesn't develop complications with nocturnal aspiration, recurrent pneumonia or bronchospasm, difficulty swallowing, or iron deficiency anemia.

REFLUX

R egurgitation

E sophageal spasm

F ood—small meals

©2002 I CAN Publishing, Inc.

L ifestyle must be modified

U se of ~~Propulsid,~~ Reglan, antacids, H_2 histamine antagonists

X out colas, milk to decrease acid production *cholate,*

ANTACIDS

Mag has had a history of an ulcer, but feels much better now since antacids coat her stomach lining. She, however, has developed another serious problem with DIARRHEA!!!! This is a major side effect of antacids containing magnesium such as Milk of Magnesia. The diarrhea must get under control or she will need to meet Alkali, a cousin, which will assist her in correcting the metabolic acidosis which may occur as a complication from the diarrhea. **Mag** should be monitored for dehydration, hypokalemia, and hyponatremia. If **Mag** were to remain on magnesium oxide for prolonged therapy, the magnesium level should be monitored periodically.

AL is also in the family and is taking an aluminum antacid such as amphogel for his ulcer symptoms. As you can see, **Al's** problem is constipation. He is so full of it that he can't get rid of it. CONSTIPATION is a major side effect of antacids containing aluminum.

Remember—Teach clients to take antacids one hour after meals and to refrain from taking other oral medications within 1-2 hours of any antacid.

AUNT ACID'S FAMILY

©1997 I CAN, Inc.

ALUMINUM　　　　**MAGNESIUM**

POSTOPERATIVE GI ASSESSMENT

Back in the operating room as a client is being prepared for abdominal surgery, drapes are used over the body to help maintain sterility. Let's use the word **DRAPES** to look at the concept of postoperative GI assessment.

D *DRESSING*–Evaluate amount and characteristics of drainage.

R *RESPIRATORY SYSTEM*–Listen for those breath sounds! Get in some T, C & DB (turning, coughing and deep breathing) to prevent atelectasis.

A *ABDOMINAL ASSESSMENT*–Watch for abdominal distention. Normal bowel sounds should be heard every 5 to 20 seconds. The abdomen should remain soft. If it becomes hard, this may indicate bleeding, paralytic ileus, or peritonitis. If in doubt, measure abdominal girth.
AMBULATE–Will decrease blood clots caused by pooling of blood in extremities. Will decrease the development of a paralytic ileus.

P *PAIN MEDICINE*–Keep them comfortable. If they have a patient-controlled analgesia (PCA) pump in place, teach them how to use it.
PATENCY OF TUBES–This can be done through irrigations and monitoring the suction of drains and tubes.

E *ELIMINATION*– Keep an I & O record.

S *SPLINT*– Splint abdominal incision during T, C, and DB.

GI ASSESSMENT

Dressing

Respiratory system

Abdominal assessment
Ambulate

Pain medicine
Patency of the tubes

Elimination

Splint

©1994 I CAN

DUMPING SYNDROME

`This is a complication that can occur after gastric resection when stomach contents enter the intestine. The image that will pull this concept together for you is the DUMP TRUCK. Imagine that you are in a dump truck on the edge of a mountain. How would you feel? We know we would be nervous as kittens, sweaty and our heart would beat very rapidly. On a mountain edge, we are sure we would be dizzy and very weak. We may also have some abdominal cramping with some distention. These signs are, of course, because we are in the **HIGH** position. (Think of TOO MUCH, TOO SOON = TOO HIGH) Too much carbohydrate, salt, liquid, refined sugar, and in the high position on top of all of that is going to make us (excuse the expression) poop! The gastric contents high in carbohydrates rapidly enter the jejunum.

To remember how to prevent this from occurring, think of the dump truck in the **LOW** position. Think LOW. Teach clients to think small (LOW) meals. The carbohydrates, salt intake, and sugar need to be LOW (small amounts). No fluids with meals or for one hour following the meal. Lie client down for 20 to 30 minutes after meals to delay stomach emptying.

DUMPING SYNDROME

As truck gets close to edge, you get nervous (sweaty, ↑pulse). You are so nervous you defecate. "Oh, poop!" (↑peristalsis, distention)

©1994 I CAN

NASOGASTRIC TUBES

First, think about tubes in general. Remember, fluid or air can flow either way in a tube. In this case, we're looking at the nasogastric tube as a feeding tube to accommodate the passing of fluid. The major safety issue with the N/G tube is PLACE-MENT. We want to know where the end of that tube is prior to putting fluid in. Nothing like dumping a feeding solution into the lung because the tube has become displaced out of the stomach! The feeding solution should be ROOM TEMPERA-TURE before putting into the body. If the client is turned to the RIGHT SIDE during the feeding, the stomach can empty better. USE GRAVITY to allow the solution to run in. Some folks use those big bulb syringes. If that's the case, squeezing the fluid in with the bulb can place undue pressure on the stomach. ASPIRATE stomach contents prior to administering a feeding. Be sure to return the gastric contents aspirated, otherwise necessary electrolytes will be wasted. Most proce-dures agree to hold the tube feeding and notify the physician if 100 cc or more are aspirated. *ENDING* the feeding with a little WATER (approximately 30–50 cc) will keep the feeding tube clean. Document this process in the chart.

NG TUBE

Never give without checking

Give warm (room temperature)

Turn to right side

Use gravity

Be sure to aspirate

End with water & chart

ANTICHOLINERGICS

The major side effects of these medications are easily seen on the next page. Some examples of these medications include: Atropine, Methantheline (Banthine), Propantheline (Pro-Banthine), and Dicyclomine hydrochloride (Bentyl). Of course these drugs are given because of the desirable effects of decreasing salivation, lacrimation, urination, diarrhea, and GI motility. Blurred vision and dilated pupils are also side effects. It's when we get too much that we get in trouble.

Remember—These medications are contraindicated in closed and open angle glaucoma, prostatic hypertrophy and obstructive bowel disease.

ANTICHOLINERGIC MEDICATIONS

Can't pee

Can't see

Can't spit

Can't shit

©1997 I CAN, Inc.

ELEVATED LIVER ENZYMES

Remembering elevated liver enzymes is as easy as **ABC**. The next page will assist you with this. When the client has a history of alcoholism, the **ast** and **alt** will be elevated. If the client has a medical problem with biliary obstruction the **alp** will be elevated. Remember there is a **p** in **alp** and he is *"plugged up Paul"*. In clients with a diagnosis of cirrhosis, the ast and alt will be elevated.

ELEVATED LIVER ENZYMES

Remember, elevated liver enzymes
are as easy as **ABC**

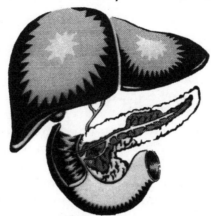

**Reprinted with permission
©1994 Creative Educators**

Alcoholism (ast, alt)

Biliary obstruction (al**p**)
"plugged up Paul"

Cirrhosis (ast, alt)

CIRRHOSIS

Here is Larry Leak Liver, who is no longer able to synthesize protein. This results in a decreased colloidal osmotic pressure. (COP holds fluid in the liver and blood vessels.) Since he no longer easily accepts blood from his unique dual blood supply, he also develops portal hypertension. This causes poor Larry to Leak fluid into the peritoneal cavity resulting in **ASCITES**. Too much swelling in the esophagus will cause Larry to get into *AIRWAY* trouble. To prevent complications from *SWELLING*, he may be started on diuretics along with potassium supplements. Salt-poor albumin will assist with hypoalbuminemia. An esophageal tamponade tube will provide compression of *BLEEDING* on esophageal *VARICES*. Prevent bleeding by soft, nonirritating foods. Let's not give him hot coffee to drink. *LABS* such as liver enzymes will be increased. Hypoalbuminemia, prolonged PT, and altered bilirubin metabolism will be seen in lab reports. Hepatic *ENCEPHALOPATHY* will result if Larry is unable to detoxify ammonia, the end product of protein metabolism. As waste products back up, Larry's *SKIN* will turn jaundiced. Decrease discomfort from pruritus. IS THERE HELP? Avoid cocktails and avoid over-the-counter drugs. Larry's liver is simply unable to detoxify them!

CIRRHOSIS

©1994 I CAN

Airway

Swelling

vari**C**es

Inspect lab work

To prevent bleeding

Encephalopathy

Skin

TYLENOL (ACETAMINOPHEN) OVERDOSE

A major undesirable effect of tylenol overdose is hepatic necrosis. It is like we have taken a hammer and beaten "the hell out of the liver." The dose of tylenol should not exceed 4g/day. Other side effects are negligible with recommended dosage. With acute poisoning, the following adverse effects may occur: **anorexia, nausea and vomiting, epigastric** or **abdominal pain, HEPATOTOXICITY, hypoglycemia,** and **hepatic coma.**

Tylenol (Acetaminophen) is a very useful drug for pain and fever. (Refer to Poison Control for more specific plans.)

Remember–Do not administer to clients with liver disease.

TYLENOL OVERDOSE

©1997 I CAN, Inc.

PANCREATITIS

After reviewing the exquisite lips on PAN AM, we feel confident that you will remember the that serum **amylase** and **lipase** are elevated in pancreatitis. **"Pancreas"** will assist you in reviewing the management for these clients.

P *PAIN MANAGEMENT* - Nonnarcotic analgesics (aspirin, ibuprofen, acetaminophen) may be tried. *PANCREATIC ENZYME* repalcement therapy may be indicated.

A *ABDOMINAL PAIN* - Typically, acute pancreatitis produces constant epigastric, periumbilical, or left or right upper abdominal pain radiating to the back, often increased by food and decreased by upright posture. Abdominal tenderness, decreased bowel sounds, distention, and fever may be part of the assessment.

N *NPO* initially - Nasogastric suction for exacerbations, Total Parental Nutrition (TPN) and fluid replacement as necessary. Initiate dietary and insulin therapy for diabetes mellitus secondary to pancreatic insufficiency.

C *CALCIUM* may be low.

R *RISK FACTORS* - Alcoholism, biliary tract disease, a penetrating duodenal ulcer and trauma are also associated with pancreatitis.

E *EVALUATE* glucose, electrolytes, hematocrit, serum amylase and lipase, hypotension, and bowel function.

A *ANALGESICS, ANTICHOLINERGICS, ANTACIDS, H2-receptor ANTAGONISTS, AND ANTIBIOTICS* are utilized.

S *STIMULANTS* such as spices, alcohol, or coffee should be avoided.

PAN AM LIPS

PAN AM

©1994 CREATIVE EDUCATORS

IN PANCREATITIS, AMYLASE AND LIPASE FLY HIGH

MENINGOCELE/
OMPHALOCELE

Both of these disorders have a sac on the outside of the body. The meningocele is a sac-like cyst of meninges filled with spinal fluid that protrudes through a defect in the bony part of the spine. A myelomeningocele is a sac-like cyst containing meninges, spinal fluid and a portion of the spinal cord with its nerves that protrudes through a defect in the vertebral column. The omphalocele is a protrusion of the intestines on the abdomen.

The nursing care is similar to a seal (**CELE**) in the water. We certainly do not want these sacs (**CELES**) to get too dry. Sterile, normal saline soaks may be used to prevent drying.

Correct positioning is also of paramount importance in preventing damage to the sac (**CELE**) as well as providing nursing care after surgery.

BE KIND TO NATURE AND
KEEP THE SEALS IN THE WATER.

Meningo<u>CELE</u>/
Omphalo<u>CELE</u>

©1994 I CAN

PIES (HYDROCEPHALUS)

Hydrocephalus is caused by an imbalance in the production and absorption of cerebral spinal fluid (CSF) in the ventricles of the brain. This infant will present with an enlarged head. Visualize **PIES** as we refer to the assessments and plans for this condition.

P *PROJECTILE VOMITING* – A symptom of increased intracranial pressure (IICP). Teach parents signs of IICP. Many of these infants are difficult to feed, so small feedings at frequent intervals are recommended.

I *IRRITABILITY* – High pitched cry is characteristic of IICP with an infant. Evaluate the level of consciousness; it is frequently the initial symptom of IICP.

E *ENLARGED HEAD AND FONTANEL* – Normally at birth, the occipital frontal circumference (OFC) is approximately 2–3 cm. larger than the chest circumference. A bulging fontanel is also a sign of IICP.
EDUCATE family and refer to appropriate community agencies.

S *SEPARATION OF SKULL* – As the CSF increases in the ventricles, there will be a separation of the cranial suture lines. They may have bulging "sunset eyes".
If infant has a **SHUNT**, observe for infection and IICP.

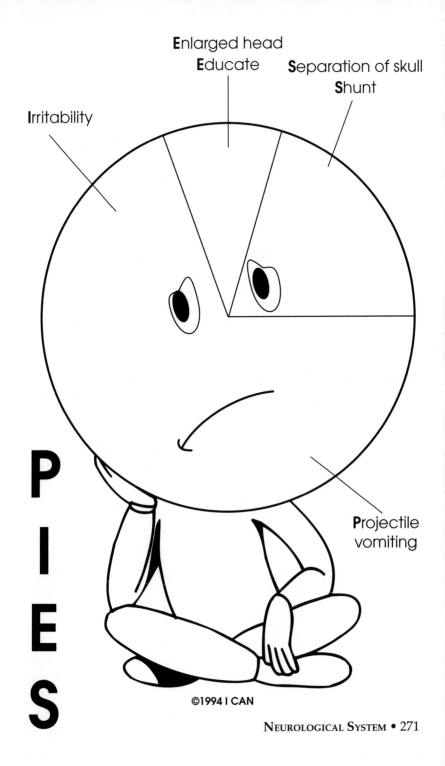

Enlarged head
Educate

Separation of skull
Shunt

Irritability

Projectile
vomiting

P
I
E
S

©1994 I CAN

GLASGOW COMA SCALE

GLASGOW COMA SCALE is often found on both nursing exams and physician orders. In the past this scale has been hard to remember, but here's help. Notice that Glasgow is running (a motor runs, indicating **MOTOR** movements in the client). See Glasgow's **EYES** are open (the client can open eyes on command). The **VERBAL** indicator, like the newspaper comics, lets you know that Glasgow is talking (the client has clear verbal ability).

The score for this scale may range from 3–15. The less responsive, the lower the score; the more responsive, the higher the score.

This is a great scale to evaluate the client's level of consciousness! In summary, the Glasgow Coma Scale evaluates motor, eye opening, and verbal ability.

GLASGOW COMA SCALE

©1994 I CAN

1. MOTOR
2. VERBAL
3. EYES OPEN

VITAL SIGNS FOR SHOCK
vs. IICP

Most of us have had the vital signs of shock drilled into our heads. We just have a hard time remembering how those vital signs change with increased intracranial pressure (IICP). Guess what? Vital signs in IICP change exactly opposite to changes in shock. All you have to remember are the vital sign changes in shock and you have the connection to recall the vital sign changes for IICP. Both shock and IICP have one commonality– both cause a loss of consciousness.

VITAL SIGNS FOR SHOCK VS. IICP

Shock	Vs.	IICP
↓	B/P	↑
↑	Pulse	↓
↑	Resp	↓
↓	Temp	↑
↓	Pulse Press	↑
↓	**LOC**	↓

NURSING CARE
FOR INCREASED
INTRACRANIAL PRESSURE

Nursing care for the clients with increased intracranial pressure is focused on decreasing the pressure and assessing the level of consciousness. For this reason we use the image of **HEADS** as a memory tool.

H *HOB*–Maintain semi-Fowler's position to promote venous drainage and respiratory function. This would be contraindicated if the client had a spinal cord injury.

E *EVALUATE NEUROLOGICAL CHECKS*–The first sign of a change in the level of intracranial pressure is an alteration in the level of consciousness. Pupils also should react equally to light.

A *AIRWAY*–Evaluate current respiratory pattern. May require intubation and control on a volume ventilator.

D *DRAINAGE*–Drainage from the ears may be cerebral spinal fluid. A CSF leak would test positive for glucose. Apply a sterile dressing over ear and evaluate for signs of meningitis.

S *SAFETY*–Seizure precautions. No sedatives or narcotics. Restrict fluids. Control temperature, and avoid coughing.

NURSING CARE FOR
↑ I C P

HO B—semi-Fowler's

Evaluate ICP

Airway

Drainage

Safety

SEIZURES

Caesar is experiencing an interruption of normal brain functioning by uncontrolled paroxysmal discharge of electrical stimuli from the neurons. **"CAESAR"** will outline the general nursing care for clients with seizures.

C *COUNSELING* is important for the family and the client to assist them in maintaining positive coping mechanisms. *CALM* - After a seizure occurs, maintain a calm atmosphere and provide privacy.

A *ANTICONVULSANTS* - Phenobarbital (Sodium luminal), Primidone (Mysoline), Carbamazepine (Tegretol), or Phenytoin (Dilantin) are some examples of anticonvulsants. *APNEA* and / or cyanosis must be monitored. Do not force anything into the client's mouth if the jaws are clenched shut. If the jaws are not clenched, place an airway in the client's mouth after the seizure. Artificial ventilation cannot be performed on a client during a tonic-clonic seizure.

E *EVALUATE* changes in the level of consciousness. After the seizure, evaluate client's orientation, activity, and any level of paralysis or muscle weakness.

S *SAFETY* - Protect the client from injuring himself by falling out of bed or striking himself on bedrails, etc. Loosen any constrictive clothing. Do not restrain client during seizure activity.

A *AVOID ALCOHOL.*
ACTIVITIES - Identify any activities that occurred immediately prior to the seizure. Describe any activity (movement) that occurred and body area affected.

R *REDUCE STIMULI.*
REMAIN with the client who is in seizure activity. Note the time the seizure began and how long it lasted. *REORIENT* client after the seizure.

Remember—SAFETY is the biggest issue.

CAESAR
(SEIZURES)

C
A
E
S
A
R

©1997 I CAN, Inc.

DILANTIN (DIAL AT TEN)

Dilane has a seizure disorder and is taking the drug dilantin. She does not feel well and is calling the nurse at 10:00 a.m. Her therapeutic level for Dilantin should be 10-20 micrograms/ml. (EASY TO REMEMBER. THERE IS A TIN (TEN) IN DILANTIN.) Her adverse reactions from this medication include **gingival hyperplasia**, (see, she's showing you her big gums) **GI disturbances, hepatotoxicity**, (her liver is visible on her abdomen) **ataxia** (her legs are shaking), **hypocalcemia** and a decrease in the absorption of **vitamin D** (the milk on the table and the sunshine coming through the window will help this problem).

If Dilane's level becomes toxic be sure and inform the physician. The medication will likely be decreased.

Remember–Teach good oral hygiene and nutrition.

liver function AST, ALT, ALP
↓
stones

DILANTIN
(DIAL AT TEN)

©1997 I CAN, Inc.

PARKINSON'S DISEASE

Meet **PARK DARK**, our little old man with Parkinson's disease. This condition results from a depletion of, or an imbalance in dopamine and increased activity in acetylcholine.

Park'S fingers want to *"PILL ROLL"* all the time. This tremor is rhythmic and rapid. Worse still, when he gets up out of the chair, his bottom is always trying to catch up with his head and never quite makes it, so he is often *ABOUT TO FALL*. *RIGIDITY* of the muscles results in jerky, uncoordinated "cogwheel" movements. Park is not always the fellow who wants to go to the restaurant for dinner because he *"KAN'T"* *SWALLOW WELL*, DROOLS his food and might get choked.

Park's last name is **Dark** because this is a dark, depressing disease, and he gets very sad about the whole thing. Medications used to enhance *DOPAMINE* secretion are levodopa (L-DOPA) and SINEMET. One of the latest drugs used for Parkinson's Disease is ropinirole (Requip), a non-ergot alkaloid dopamine agonist. *ARTANE* and cogentin are used to decrease effects of acetylcholine. Sometimes *COFFEE RESTRICTION* can reduce the pill rolling. Some ANTIHISTAMINES may be helpful to *KEEP MUSCLE TREMORS DOWN*.

PARK DARK bears watching. He unfortunately falls, spills hot food on himself and can get depressed to the point of harming himself. *He will need your support!*

PARK DARK

Pill rolling

About to fall

Rigidity

Kan't swallow/speak (drools)

Dopamine/L-Dopa/Sinemet

Artane—improves rigidity

Restrict coffee

Keep tremors down with
   antihistimine

©1994 I CAN

MYASTHENIA GRAVIS

Why didn't somebody tell us that myasthenia gravis means grave muscle weakness? If they had, we would have asked ourselves where are the muscles? The heart is a muscle. Muscles help move the chest for breathing and the legs for walking, to name just a few. If there is grave muscle weakness, we can see why **MYRA DYSTONIA** will get into deep trouble fast if she doesn't get her muscle strengthening medication (prostigmin or mestinon) on TIME! As you can see **MYRA DYSTONIA** has drooping eyelids and may even experience some difficulty moving her face. She will NOT have any sensory deficit, loss of reflexes, or muscle atrophy. This progressive weakness is caused from a failure in transmission of nerve impulses due to acetylcholine release. There are no cures at the present time. **"TIME"** is one of the most important factors.

T *TENSILON* is a drug with a short half life that will strengthen muscle weakness in Myra. This makes it a good drug for DIAGNOSIS and differentiating types of crisis (cholinergic crisis versus myasthenic crisis). It is not routinely given for treatment due to its short term effect.

I *INFECTION* and exercise make MYRA worse.

M *MUST* give medications on time. We sure don't want MYRA to go on that ventilator. We MUST avoid the use of sedatives and tranquilizers which cause respiratory depression. We MUST not give the client anything to eat or drink during a myasthenic crisis due to the risk of aspiration. After the crisis, remember to assess the ability to swallow and give a diet which is soft and easily swallowed.

E *EXACERBATIONS* and remission are part of this experience, but since the weakness is progressive it's likely to get worse with TIME.

MYRA DYSTONIA

Tensilon

Infection

Meds on time

Exacerbations

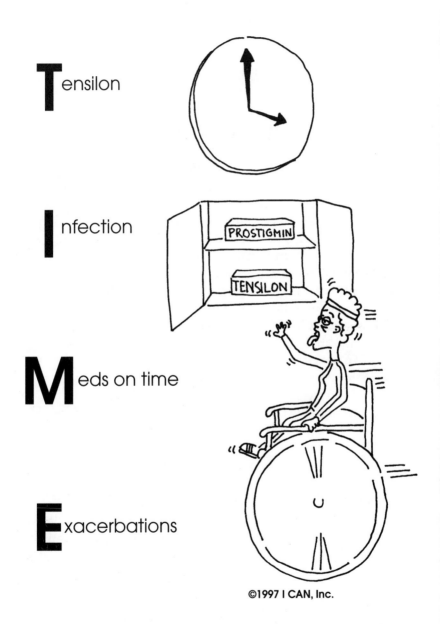

©1997 I CAN, Inc.

BELL'S PALSY

Ring the Bell for the Palsy that affects the seventh cranial nerve, resulting in muscle flaccidity on one side of the face. If the facial appearance is permanent, clients may need counseling assistance with maintaining a positive *IMAGE*. They may be ringing your call bell because of "pain" behind the ear, drooping of the mouth and an eyelid that won't close. *ANAL-GESICS* will be given to decrease the pain behind the ear. Ophthalmic ointment and eye patches may be needed at night to prevent drying of the cornea on the affected side. During the day, instilling *METHYLCELLULOSE* drops will help keep the eye moist (*GIVE EYE CARE*). Due to the discomfort, *EVALUATE* the client's *ABILITY TO EAT*.

Treatment may consist of corticosteroids and vasodilators. An inability to close the eyelid on the affected side, and a sagging mouth is scary; however, proper treatment and good nursing care will usually help clear up the problem with little residual.

BELL'S PALSY

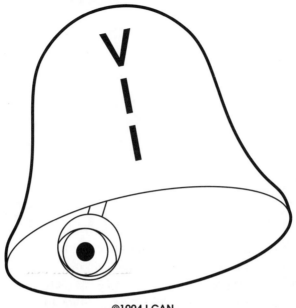

©1994 I CAN

I mage

M ethylcellulose

A nalgesics *nerve #7*

G ive eye care

E valuate ability to eat

TRIGEMINAL NEURALGIA

This is a cranial nerve disorder affecting the sensory branches of the trigeminal nerve (cranial nerve V). Let us introduce you to Luke W. Arm. Luke says, "Hot food is painful!" He has a closed eye from frequent blinking and tearing. Facial twitching and grimacing are characteristic. The pain he experiences is usually brief and ends as abruptly as it begins. The word "**PAINE**" will help you remember the nursing care for Luke W. Arm.

The medical management of pain may be Dilantin or Tegretol. The surgical intervention is a local nerve block or interruption of the nerve impulse transmission.

TRIGEMINAL NEURALGIA

P ain is excruciating

A void hot or cold

I ncrease protein and calories

N erve, cranial V

E ye care

©1994 I CAN

ADVERSE EFFECTS OF IMMOBILITY

It is **AWFUL** being immobilized! Have you ever tried it? The nursing goals are to prevent these potential complications from occurring.

A *ATELECTASIS*–There may be a decrease in client's ability to cough and move those secretions which will result in a decreased oxygen exchange. Infections can lead to this complication. Encourage turning, coughing and deep breathing. Putting the head of the bed up will help with breathing and coughing. Maintain adequate hydration.

W *WASTING OF THE BONES*–Demineralization of bones leads to muscle weakness and atrophy. Range of motion exercises are mandatory. Maintain appropriate alignment while positioning.

F *FUNCTION LOSS*–This can result from the above problem. Prevent by active contracting and relaxing large muscles.

U *URINARY STASIS*–Increase those fluids and decrease the calcium intake. If possible, have client sit to void.

L *LAST BUT NOT LEAST CONSTIPATION*–Encourage diet with adequate protein, bulk and liquids.

IMMOBILITY

Atelectasis

Wasting of bones

Functional loss of muscle

Urinary stasis

Last but not least, constipation

©1994 I CAN

PERIPHERAL VASCULAR DISEASE

	V	*VENOUS VALVES DEFECTIVE*
		VEIN WALLS LEAK
		VARICOSE VEINS
	E	*ELEVATE LEGS*
W	E	*IGHT REDUCTION*
BRAW	N	*Y IN COLOR*
H	O	*SE*
T	O	*PICAL STEROIDS*
	U	*ULCERS*
	S	*STANDING A LOT!*
		SKIN COLOR CHANGES

PERIPHERAL VASCULAR DISEASE

ALLOPURINOL (ZYLOPRIM)

Allopurinol (Zyloprim) the drug of choice to prevent **GOUT** decreases uric acid synthesis. Uric acid is the end product of purine metabolism. Condition of hyperuricemia may also occur in individuals receiving chemotherapy (secondary gout). Medications for an acute attack may include colchicine, indomethacin (Indocin) or naproxen (Naprosyn).

Gout is generally rapid with swelling and a painful joint. Typically the uric acid crystals are in the large toe, but may also involve ankles and knees. During an acute attack, protect the affected joint by immobilizing the joint. Encourage gradual weight reduction. Instruct the client to avoid salicylates. Encourage **high fluid intake** (>3L / day) to increase excretion of uric acid and to prevent the development of uric acid stones.

Teach clients to avoid foods high in purines such as **organ meats**, shell fish, and preserved fish (anchovies, sardines) and avoid **alcohol**. We would like to see the urine **output increased** to 2 liters per day to help decrease the risk of stones. Clients at risk for stones may be given trisodium citrate for urine alkalinization.

Remember–Clients with renal insufficiency should receive a reduced dose of Allopurinol.

ALLOPURINOL (GOUT)

Gulp 3 liters fluid per day

Ø organ meats or wines

Urine output increased to 2 liters per day

Teach

©1997 I CAN, Inc.

OSTEOPOROSIS

JOSEPHINE BONE-A-PART is working to prevent immobility in her "mature years". She is on a treadmill because weight-bearing exercise increases bone strength. She is taking her Fosomax, Calcium, and Estrogen to decrease her risk of developing osteoporosis. She knows that her drinking and smoking have got to stop if she doesn't want to be laid up with broken **BONES.**

B *BONE* density studies are the noninvasive x-ray diagnostic tests that are commonly used. There is no prep, no pain and not much time involved in this x-ray. Just lie down and they'll shoot it.

O *OUT* of calcium is an issue. Inadequate calcium intake early in life may have predisposed Josephine Bone-A-Part to the development of osteoporosis. Calcium supplemental therapy (about 1500mg per day) is usually recommended for post-menopausal women. Young women should be advised to have a daily dietary intake of at least 1000 to 1500 mg of calcium per day. Magnesium and Vitamin D may also need to be supplemented.

N *NEED FOSOMAX* **AFTER** osteoporosis has developed. This drug aides the BONES to become more calcified, stronger and denser. To keep down the GI side effects of this medication, drink with 8 ounces of water first thing in the morning. Stay sitting up and NPO for at least half an hour before eating or taking other drugs. Yep, it's a pain!

E *ESTROGEN* given orally has demonstrated its ability to decrease the incidence of osteoporosis. In addition, estrogen improves the client's lipid profile (HDL cholesterol rises, LDL cholesterol falls) and overall cardiovascular risk declines. Weight bearing EXERCISE, such as walking, helps the BONES. EDUCATION early in life will assist in preventing complications from osteoporosis.

S *STRESS* fractures especially of the hip, waist or vertebra are common. Education and prevention of falls are important in minimizng fractures and maintaining independence for post-menopausal women.

Remember–Prevention is the BEST action!

JOSEPHINE BONE-A-PART

©1997 I CAN, Inc.

ARTHRITIS

Arthur has osteoarthritis. He wakes up in the morning stiff and achy and finds it hard to reach his walking cane. His fingers are all swollen at the joints (Herberden's nodules) and other joints are affected. He may feel better after his shower as the hot water warms up those joints. Arthur has on his swim trunks because he is going to water therapy at the local spa. Water therapy is probably the best exercise since it better protects his weight bearing joints. He will definitely need to rest after his swim.

Tylenol may be the medication of choice and Arthur will have to be reminded to keep his dosage at or below 4 gms/24 hours to prevent an overdose. (See **TYLENOL OVERDOSE**)

Remember–Arthur may not want to move because of his pain, but physical activity is imperative for him to retain his independence.

ARTHUR ITIS

NONSTEROIDAL ANTI-INFLAMMATORY DRUGS (NSAIDs)

NSAIDs are a group of medications that prevent prostaglandin synthesis. What does that mean? Prostaglandins contribute to the following: inflammation, body temperature, pain transmission, platelett aggregation, and other actions. These prostaglandins are not stored, but are released on demand.

What type of physical problems may benefit from NSAIDs? Fever and inflammation (ie. arthritis) can be reduced by these medications.

Are there any undesirable effects from NSAIDs? There are several undesirable effects that the nurse must assess and educate clients to report. These include GI upset or bleeding, **ototoxicity** (ringing in the ears), **hepatic necrosis**, or **nephritis**.

As a nurse, what should be included in the plan of care?

1. Administer medications with **food to decrease GI irritation.**

2. Teach clients about actions and side effects and report any dark, tarry stools, "coffee ground or bloody emesis", other **GI distress** or **ringing in the ears.**

3. Instruct client to inform health care providers about these medications prior to any dental or other type of surgery. NSAIDs should be discontinued approximately 5–7 days before the procedure to prevent any complications with bleeding.

4. NSAIDs are not the drugs of choice if the client has any compromise in either the renal system or the liver.

5. Evaluate the effectiveness of the NSAIDs.

NSAIDs

No alcohol

Side effects

Aspirin sensitivity—
do not give

Ibuprofen, Indocin are
a few examples

Do take with food

©1997 I CAN, Inc.

Stop 5–7 days before surgery

CARE OF CLIENT IN TRACTION

Ellie Elephant gets in more trouble. She has fallen, **FRAC-TURED** her trunk, and is in traction. We will need a *FIRM MATTRESS*, and will probably need help putting her through *RANGE OF MOTION* exercises. Pay attention to those feet; we don't want a problem with *FOOT DROP*. Without good body *ALIGNMENT*, Ellie may get contractures and decubiti. *ALIGNMENT* will also help keep the traction pulling from both ends which is the reason for traction anyway. Let's get Ellie a *TRAPEZE*, so that she can help us turn her to keep the pneumonia away. Ellie needs to cough and deep breathe on regular intervals to prevent *RESPIRATORY COMPLICA-TIONS*. One *COMPLICATION* of a fracture of long bones is a fat embolism. It can be transported to the lungs producing symptoms of acute *RESPIRATORY* distress. Now what will we do about her *URINARY retention*? Increase fluid intake. Ellie may need help with the bedpan. Be sure and *evaluate for circulatory impairments*. The 5 P's will help. They are pain, pallor of skin, pulses (especially distal to the injury), paresthesia, and paralysis. Compartmental syndrome can be a major problem.

Good Luck! Elephants and people in traction can be a major challenge!

CARE OF CLIENT IN TRACTION

Firm mattress
 oot drop

ROM—for unaffected
    extremities

Alignment

Complications

Trapeze

Urinary retention

©1994 I CAN

Respiratory complications

Evaluate circulatory
   impairments
            (5 P's)

CRUTCH WALKING

Remembering how to instruct the client to use crutches while walking up and down the stairs is "INSANELY EASY". Just look at our friend, Charlie, with his crutches on the next page. He is putting his good leg up on the stair first "UP TO HEAVEN"! When he goes down, his bad leg will go first! Remember, "BAD GOES TO YOU KNOW WHERE".

CRUTCH WALKING

CARE OF THE SPINAL CORD CLIENT

"**CRUTCHES THE COLLIE**" dog has been out partying with the neighborhood dogs and has been in an automobile accident. He broke his neck and is unfortunately paralyzed from the neck down. The paramedic dog who came to the scene had to access his airway by a "jaw thrust" and log roll him to stabilize his neck. This will minimize further **CORD DAMAGE**. Assess Collie's breath sounds and signs of hypoxia. Incentive spirometry and chest physiotherapy will assist in optimizing **RESPIRATORY FUNCTION**. Due to his loss of bladder function, **URINARY** retention is a problem. He will either have an indwelling catheter or require intermittent catheterization. Prevent urinary tract infections! Because Collie is immobile watch for blood clots (**THROMBUS**). Compression stockings may help venous return. **CARDIOVASCULAR STABILITY** can be a problem due to **SHOCK** or autonomic dysreflexia. (Refer to **AUTONOMIC DYSREFLEXIA**.)

Collie needs a **NEURO ASSESSMENT** for IICP (Refer to IICP visual). **FLUIDS AND ROUGHAGE** are necessary to keep bladder and bowels working. Calories and protein need to be increased. Watch for **SKIN BREAKDOWN**. An ounce of prevention is worth a pound of cure. Collie is going to have a major life change. He will need **SUPPORT** in ventilating his feelings and establishing realistic short-term goals.

CARE OF
SPINAL CORD CLIENT

C ord damage

R espiratory function

U rinary and bowel function

T hrombus

C ardiovascular stability

H elp maintain ongoing
neurological assessment

E ncourage adequate
fluid and nutrition

S kin breakdown
hock
upport

ANTICOAGULANTS

Coumadin and Heparin are used to inhibit thrombus and clot formation. They chip away at the clot to make it smaller. Clotting times will be prolonged which will assist in maintaining the flow or "stream of blood."

The key to successfully remembering the lab reports and antidotes for the appropriate anticoagulants are to think of (H) looking like 2 tt's in Heparin. The lab report necessary to evaluate while clients are on heparin is Ptt. The antidote also has 2 t's in it (protamine sulfate).

Coumadin's antidote is vitamin K. **C** and **K** sound alike which will help with association. The lab report which needs to be monitored is Pt.

Labs now report INR (international normalized ratio) values. The range for most clients on anticoagulants is 2–3. The exceptions are mechanical heart valves and recurrent thromboembolism clients who should be anticoagulated to an INR of 3–4.5.

ANTICOAGULANTS

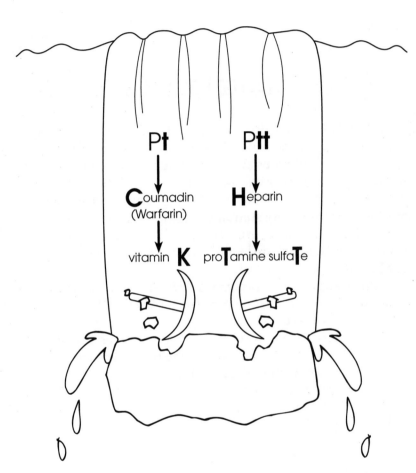

©1997 I CAN, Inc.

AUTONOMIC DYSREFLEXIA

This condition may occur in clients with a spinal cord injury at T_6 or higher. The stimuli below the level of injury triggers the sympathetic nervous system to dump catecholamines resulting in hypertension. Spinal injury blocks the normal transmission of sensory impulses. There is an exaggerated response to the sensory stimuli.

The most common causes are the 3 F's: *FULL BLADDER, FECAL IMPACTION,* and a *FUNNY FEELING WITH THE SKIN.*

The assessments that occur as a result of these causes are: *FLUSHING and DIAPHORESIS, HEADACHE, HYPERTEN-SION,* and *BRADYCARDIA.* The priority treatment is to identify and REMOVE the CAUSE. Frequently the dysreflexia will subside. If possible, the head of the bed can be elevated. Watch the hypertension, so that it doesn't get out of hand. These folks feel real bad and usually cannot tell you their problem. Once their bladder or bowel is emptied the sweating and bad feelings go away.

AUTONOMIC DYSREFLEXIA
(Injuries at T$_6$ or higher)

Causes

   1.**F**ull bladder

   2.**F**ecal impaction

   3.**F**unny feeling with the skin

Assessments

   1.Flushing & Diaphoresis

   2.Headache

   3.Hypertension

   4.Bradycardia

MAGIC 2's

The magician is pulling the prescription drugs out of his magic hat and reminding you that you can use the "MAGIC 2's" as a way to remember the toxicity level. These are the medications most commonly monitored for therapeutic dosage.

Monitoring Drugs By The Magic 2's

Drug	Range	Toxicity
Digitalis	.5-1.5	**2**
Lithium	.6-1.2	**2**
Aminophylline (Theophylline)	10-20	**20**
Dilantin	10-20	**20**
Acetaminophen	1-30	**200**

©1997 I CAN, Inc.

THE MAGIC 4's

Sometimes it's hard to remember those electrolyte extracellular levels; however, we MUST because they affect the heart as recorded by the EKG. The digit **4** can be magic in helping to remember. Even though not electrolytes, the hemoglobin and hematocrit can also be remembered using a **4**. For example if the hemoglobin is 14 the hematocrit will be 42. The pH, pCO_2, and HCO_3, may also be difficult to remember until you review the **MAGIC 4's**.

The Magic 4's

Electrolyte	Range	Magic 4
K	3.5–5.5	**4**
Cl	98–106	104
Na	135–145	140
pH	7.34–7.45	7.40
pCO_2	35–45	40
HCO_3	22–26	24

A good way to remember the Hct is: 3 x Hb (10-14)

INDEX

Note: Page numbers in italics refer to images.

People learn in many different ways. We want to tell you about our stuff because our business is to help you PASS.
www.icanpublishing.com

NURSING MADE INSANELY EASY, 3rd Ed. is a pocket-sized book, chock full of drawings and information streamlining nursing and allied health education with an EASY totally different bottom line approach to concepts.

E essential concepts assist learners to prepare for exams, exit exams, and NCLEX®.

A assist nursing graduates to remember health and disease concepts.

S special images per page with essential concepts on the opposite page.

Y your learning is memorable and fun.

For example, one look at "Go Getter Gertrude" and you will remember the most important facts about the concept of hyperthyroidism and Graves' Disease _forever_.

NCLEX-RN™: 101 HOW TO PASS 3rd Ed.
Helps you **FOCUS** on your success!

F feel more confident
O omit surprises on NCLEX-RN™
C cut through piles of notes
U use to pinpoint your study needs
S see yourself improve

The book has over 800 critical thinking questions based on nursing behaviors that are the backbone of the NCLEX-RN™ exam. It comes with a CD that is a sample exam containing practice questions for you to practice before "test day".

NCLEX-RN™ REVIEW audio tapes. Pass your NCLEX® with confidence after these fun and easy listening audio tapes. These tapes are of an actual live review course that includes the concepts listed in the NCLEX-RN® test plan. The NURSING MADE INSANELY EASY book comes with this set of 7 tapes. We CAN help you prepare for the NCLEX® and you can listen at your convenience!

NCLEX-RN® non-traditional live review, brought to your site for 50 participants or more or call our office 1-800-234-0575 for information and dates on our sites in more than 15 states. The NCLEX® exam did not get harder just different. This course provides the SECRETS to NCLEX success in a fun and easy 3 day format. The books NURSING MADE INSANELY EASY, 3rd ed. and NCLEX-RN ™ 101: HOW TO PASS, 4th ed. with a CD of a sample exam accompanying the book are included in the cost of this review course.

A YEAR OF WEEKLY DEVOTIONALS

FINDING JOY
in Jesus

Available on Amazon
https://www.amazon.com/dp/B079VTNMY9

Prayer Journals also Available on Amazon

https://www.amazon.com/dp/1693027763

https://www.amazon.com/dp/0578633906